Children's Fears

by Dr. Benjamin B. Wolman

GROSSET & DUNLAP
A FILMWAYS COMPANY

Publishers • New York

Contents

CONTENTS

CONTENTS

Preface

Forty years ago I got my first job as a child psychologist in an institution for problem children overseas. A few years later I was appointed director of a child guidance center where I worked with parents and their children. During World War II, I was in charge of a network of psychological services for families of servicemen, and supervised individual, group, and family therapy for wives, parents, and other family members of enlisted men. Since then, I have written and edited several books for my colleagues, and have been uninterruptedly involved in clinical practice, teaching, supervision, and research in child psychology.

The present book is for parents. Part One, Psychology of Children's Fears, systematically describes the origin and nature of fears (Chapter I) and the developmental aspects of children's fears (Chapters II–VII). Chapter VIII offers guidance for parents. Part Two describes children's fears in alphabetical order. Each section is followed by a brief suggestion to parents and educators.

Fears are part of every child's growth and development, and children should be helped to outgrow their infantile fears and to become mature adults. Mature and well-adjusted adults are not fearless, but their fears are rational, and they can successfully cope with them. They are reasonably cautious and avoid unnecessary risks, and they are reasonably self-assured. They neither fear nonexisting dangers nor overlook real ones.

Certain childhood experiences help children to become well-adjusted adults, while other experiences may prevent their growth and even cause regression.

The developmental approach of this book will help parents view their children's fears in proper perspective—what is normal at one age may be abnormal at another age. Parental guidance must be geared to the child's growth and development. There is no reason to push a child to be more mature than he can be or expect him to do now what he will eventually accomplish at a later stage. On the other hand, parental overprotectiveness may unduly slow down or even harm the normal process of growth.

One cannot make a tree grow—growth is a natural process and a seed must go through certain developmental stages before it develops into a sapling and then a tree. A good gardener watches the process and creates the best possible conditions. Parents have no more power than gardeners. The aim of this book is to help them apply their love and common sense wisely.

The idea for this book was suggested by Mr. Douglas Corcoran, editor at Grosset & Dunlap. I am profoundly indebted to him, and to Mr. Robert Markel, Editor-in-Chief of Grosset & Dunlap, for cordial encouragement and competent editorial advice.

BENJAMIN B. WOLMAN

How to
Use This Book

This book is divided into two parts. Part One describes fears in systematic developmental order. Part Two describes children's fears in alphabetical order. You will get the most out of this book if you read it from beginning to end. However, if you are interested in a general understanding of fears read:

Chapter I

If you are interested in the relationship between children's fears and child development read:

Chapter II

If you want to know about fears related to a particular age read:

Chapter III for the first year of life
Chapter IV for the second year of life
Chapter V for years three through five

HOW TO USE THIS BOOK

Chapter VI for years six through eleven
Chapter VII for adolescence

If you want to know about the role of parents read:

Chapter VIII

If you are interested in a particular fear, look up the fear you are concerned with, which appears in alphabetical order in Part Two, starting on page 103.

Part One
Psychology of
Children's Fears

Chapter I.
Fear, Anxiety, and Courage

Fear and Survival

All living creatures fight for survival, and the emotion of fear is one of the most important self-preservation mechanisms in humans and animals. It is a most useful warning signal: "Watch out, someone or something is going to hurt you. If you think you are strong enough to overcome the threatening person or animal, get ready to fight. If the threat is too great for you, seek cover, run for your life." Fear provides the necessary motivation for mobilizing one's energies and acting cautiously and prudently.

Fearless people would not survive very long. They would cross streets on red lights and be run over by cars. They would lean out of open windows, lose their balance, and end up on the pavement. They would not hesitate to start a fight with ferocious beasts and armed robbers. They would carelessly throw burning matches on curtains and taste poisons.

The greatest fear, the archfear, is the fear of death. All living organisms react with fear to threats to their life. They respond in a variety of ways, but whatever they do has one aim, common to the entire animal world: *survival.*

Some organisms are better equipped to fight off threats to their life because they have stronger muscles, quicker legs, sharper teeth and claws; they are physically stronger. Other organisms are better equipped to outsmart their enemies; they are more intelligent and mentally more alert and stronger.

Power

Power is the ability to survive, and the possession of power is the main determinant of survival. Death is the nadir of power; omnipotence is the summit. Every human being has some ammount of power, be it physical, mental, political, financial, or some other kind. Power is the ability to satisfy one's needs, and survival is the common name of all needs. In order to survive, people need oxygen, water, food, shelter, protection against enemies, and so on. The more pwoer they have, the better their chances for survival. The use of power extends beyond fundamental biological needs, and artistic powerful individuals are able to satisfy their cultural and artistic needs and follow their personal ambitions and desires. They have the power to live well.

The more one is aware of the extent and limitations of one's power, the better use one can make of one's resources. Some people overestimate their power, others underestimate it. Those who overestimate their power take unnecessary and costly risks; those who underesti-

PSYCHOLOGY OF CHILDREN'S FEARS

mate it don't try for what they could safely attain but prefer to live cowardly on the margin of life.

I have come across both types of people in my psychotherapeutic practice. In my book *Victims of Success* (pp. 15–16) I described two patients, one who overestimated his financial power and one who underestimated it:

> ˙ Mr. Gold [who drove a brand-new Cadillac] wanted to "impress" people by his conspicuous consumption. He hoped to cover up his rather modest income and feeling of inferiority by giving the impression of being a millionaire, which he was not. He was spending more money than his financial position justified; in restaurants and when traveling, he gave more than generous tips, acting as if his life and status were dependent upon the approval of waiters, taxi-drivers, doormen, and porters.
>
> On the other hand, some people tend to hold onto their money as if it were their last dime. Mr. Clark . . . had a chauffeur-driven limousine at his disposal; but whenever the limousine was unavailable, he took a bus or the subway. Even when he knew he might be late for our appointment, Mr. Clark could not persuade himself to "splurge" on a taxicab. This highly intelligent man, whose logical mind contributed greatly to the success of [his] company, often displayed unreasonable frugality, bordering on pettiness: buying cheap shirts and ties, wearing old clothes, and (when he believed no one saw him) eating frankfurters for lunch. Mr. Gold, on the contrary, smoked expensive cigars, wore expensive, custom-tailored suits, and always volunteered to pick up the tab for others.
>
> Normal people spend their money judiciously; exhibitionists spend more than they can afford; misers are afraid to part with what they have.

Money is merely one source of power, though a very important one in our society. One can also increase one's

CHILDREN'S FEARS

power by improving one's physical fitness, muscular strength, and agility. This makes one feel better equipped for physical confrontations. Power has always attracted people, and children are fascinated by such characters as Samson and Hercules. Little children like to wrestle. Often they wonder who is stronger, the leopard or the crocodile, the rhinoceros or the elephant. Grade-school children love rough games, and many preadolescents and adolescents like to show off their physical strength and agility.

Cunning and weaponry are main sources of power and security. People have always aspired to political power, leadership and control of others, and history is full of men and women who strove to accumulate power, wealth, and glory.

Acceptance

The desire to be strong is universal, and people derive a great deal of satisfaction from the feeling of power. However, no human being is so powerful that he can overcome all threats, and no one with a sober mind believes he is omnipotent. Some anxious people try to vanquish their painful feelings of weakness by morbidly seeking a temporary, misleading, and harmful escape in alcohol and drugs. Well-adjusted individuals do not seek such illusory escapes from weakness. They put all their efforts into increasing their real *power* and *security;* that is, awareness of their power.

There are two rational methods of increasing one's power: one is by a realistic growth of power and the other is by forming alliances. Both methods increase one's chances for survival. The first method implies depending on one's own resources; the second, depending on others. Power and security can be substantially increased through interaction with other people. Not all types of interaction, however, are conducive to security, for people perceive one another in two dimensions: *power* and *acceptance.*

Power means the ability to satisfy needs. The concept of power includes physical strength, intelligence, experience, competence, and so on. In short, it represents whatever people need to survive and to make the best of their lives.

In civilized societies power is diversified and distributed among a great many people. When we are sick, the physician has the power to cure us. When we are in legal trouble, the lawyer can help us. The peak of power is omnipotence, which no human being can possess. If a vertical line is drawn to reflect the amount of power people can possess, the top of the line is omnipotence and death is the bottom.

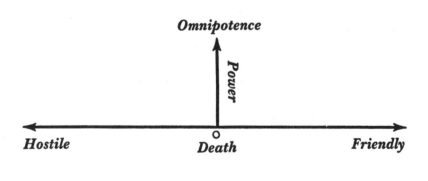

Power can be used to help or to hurt, to protect life or to destroy it. The way power is used represents the dimension of *acceptance,* which can be positive or negative. Positive acceptance (friendliness) means willingness to use one's power to help, to care and protect; negative acceptance (hostility) means willingness to use one's power to hurt and destroy.

People react to situations and to other people in accordance with their perception—that is, the way they see them. They seek the help of a dentist they perceive as *strong* (competent and capable of taking care of their teeth) and *friendly* (honest, sincere, and willing). They do not choose a dentist they perceive as *weak* (incompetent) or *hostile* (dishonest and deceitful). Though they may err in their perceptions—overestimate or underestimate people or misconstrue things—it is important to remember that people respond not to what is but to what they see. Of course, the more mature a person is, the more able he is to check and validate his perceptions. The ability to distinguish between wish and truth is called *reality testing*.

When people meet, they usually size each other up in terms of power and acceptance, power meaning the ability to satisfy needs, acceptance meaning the willingness to do so. Normally, people seek to be associated with individuals they perceive as both strong and friendly. Human relations are determined by power and acceptance *as* perceived by individuals.

There are four determinants of human relations, two related to power, namely strong or weak, and two related to acceptance, namely friendly or hostile.

Strong and friendly people elicit respect, admiration, and the desire to associate with them. We tend to follow them as leaders for they can be trusted (acceptance) and depended on (power). We seek to be allied with them and cooperate with them, and we do not wish to lose their valuable friendship.

PSYCHOLOGY OF CHILDREN'S FEARS

Strong and hostile people elicit fear and hatred. We try to avoid them and, whenever the opportunity arises, to hurt them.

Weak and friendly people elicit pity. We do not respect them nor do we care what they think of us. We may, however, feel sorry for them and help them.

Weak and hostile people elicit disgust and hatred, and we may wish to hurt them.

There are two main sources of security, and two main ways of combating fears: one's own power and the power of faithful and dependable allies (acceptance).

Dependence on one's power is *self-reliance;* dependence on strong and friendly allies is *trust.* Self-confidence and trust are the two main factors in combating one's fears and achieving security. In adults, self-reliance is paramount. Children, having rather limited power, must depend on parents or parental substitutes. This trust in loving and protecting parents, and their own growth, will gradually enable them to reach maturity. *The road from infancy to adulthood is the road from dependence to self-reliance.*

Fear and Adjustment

Fear is a self-preservation signal that mobilizes the physiological resources of the organism. It speeds up the heartbeat and blood pressure, increases the supply of necessary sugar, and activates the secretion of adrenalin and noradrenalin. The anterior lobe of the pituitary gland and the adrenal medulla increase their secretions, which improves the individual's ability to cope with danger by fight or flight. Physical strength and speed of movement are augmented, so the entire organism is in a state of alert mobilization.

There is no evidence that these physiological changes

are accompanied by increases in perceptual ability, rational judgment, and speed of reasoning, although an anticipation of future consequences sometimes improves mental functioning. The physiological reactions to fear that mobilize physical energies are exceedingly useful to animals, but since human beings can rarely solve their problems by sheer physical force or by running away from them, there is no clear-cut evidence that these reactions are very useful to us.

A threat may incite one to fight or flight. In adult animals, especially males, a threat provokes an attack on the source of threat. Additional factors, such as hunger, absence of escape routes, and familiarity with the territory, encourage aggression. Infant animals and sick or tired animals tend to escape.

Human beings, especially in early childhood, often react impulsively to threatening stimuli. A totally innocent loud noise produced by a nearby firecracker can elicit a startle. As children grow, they develop a mental control apparatus and, unless totally taken by surprise, they react to threats in a more mature and rational way.

An adult organism reacts in a selective and purposeful manner to threatening stimuli. We blow out a burning match, put a bandage on a scratched finger, and open an umbrella in the rain, but we do not run for our lives in any of these minor emergencies.

The human brain at birth is not capable of selectively reacting to stimuli and controlling the behavior of the organism. Oncoming stimuli elicit *mass reaction,* and the total organism responds to a situation that could be handled by a slight motion of a hand or leg. It takes a good deal of maturation before the child learns to chase away a mosquito with the motion of a hand and not burst into tears.

The reaction of an adult organism to a stimulus resembles a well-tuned piano: You press a certain key, and the piano responds with an appropriate tone. An infant's reaction resembles a disorganized piano: you touch one key, and you hear several other, unrelated tones.

A threatening situation can evoke fear or anger or both, depending on how one perceives the source of threat. Strong and hostile enemies elicit more fear, weak and hostile ones, more anger. Fear and anger are two sides of the coin of self-preservation. Fear leads to flight, anger to fight. One reacts with fear when one believes that the threatening forces are too much to cope with. One reacts with anger when one feels one can defeat the hostile forces.

Both fear and anger are hostile reactions to hostile stimuli. The weaker a person is, the more prone he or she is to react in this manner. A self-assured mother does not feel hostile toward a cranky, angry, difficult child because he does not represent a threat to her. She disarms him and calms him down by her calm and friendly attitude, for the bigger and stronger one is, the more magnanimous one can be.

A little child is weak and therefore prone to fear and anger. He does not know how to cope with angry parents; their anger and overwhelming power elicit fear and help-less anger from him, which is definitely maladjustive (see Chapter VIII, Do's and Don'ts for Parents).

Fear and Perception

Human behavior is guided not by things as they are but by things as they seem. A person may have power and many friends, and be unaware of these facts. Power and acceptance as *perceived* by the individual are the true determinants of his behavior. An individual who is aware of his own power and of his allies has no irrational fears, and is better prepared to cope with threats that must be feared.

CHILDREN'S FEARS

An overestimation of one's own resources combined with an underestimation of potential threats leads to a maladjustive lack of fear. A carefree, cocksure, unsuspecting attitude is self-defeating. On the other hand, an underestimation of one's own power and an overestimation of threats increases one's fears and limits one's ability to cope rationally with danger.

Fear is normal and helps one to survive provided it is *realistic* and based on an accurate evaluation of the potential threat and one's own power. Fear is adjustive if it corresponds to the real situation. For instance, fear of a cobra, of vicious beasts, or of a stormy ocean is normal, but fear of ants, of a little puppy, or of a toilet flush is irrational and maladjustive.

When one is stronger than the potential threat, there is no reason to fear. When one is weaker than the threatening force, fear is useful. Thus fear is rational when it is based on the awareness of overwhelming threats, but irrational when it is grounded in an overestimation of the threatening forces and/or an underestimation of one's own powers. Overestimation of his own powers makes a person foolhardy and vulnerable, but underestimation makes him fear insignificant or nonexisting dangers.

Fears based on a realistic assessment of danger in comparison to one's own and one's allies' power are useful and adjustive. Fear of crossing streets on the red light is realistic, for cars move faster than people. This fear saves lives. So does the fear of stormy oceans, forest fires, and armed gangsters, unless one is especially well equipped to overcome these dangers.

There is a positive correlation between realistic fears and intelligence. Bright children are usually earlier and better aware of potential dangers than dull ones, and as they grow older, they overcome irrational fears more rapidly than less intelligent children. Some fears, like the fear of loss of balance, of fast-approaching objects, of sudden and loud noises, do not require any intelligence; they are innate. But the fear of putting fingers into an electric outlet, or of playing with sharp scissors, or of crossing the street on a red light is not innate, and an intelligent child faster comprehends the potential dangers than a less intelligent one. An intelligent child is more likely to be cautious because he is capable of anticipating potential dangers. The more intelligent a child is, the faster he becomes aware of real dangers and learns to distinguish them from imaginary ones. A bright child begins to question the existence of goblins and spooks because he is better able to think logically than a dull child (see Section 48.)

Fear and Maladjustment

Alarm signals do not always elicit appropriate reactions. Instead of mobilizing one's physical and mental resources for fight or flight, fear can have a paralyzing effect and substantially reduce one's chances for survival.

Acute states of fear can elicit counterproductive physiological reactions such as trembling, profuse perspiration, faint feelings, weakness in joints and muscles, nausea, diarrhea, and disturbances in motor coordination. The severely frightened individual may seek escape when none is needed.

Exaggerated fears can have a crippling effect on human behavior. People obsessed by fears live on the margin of life, fearing to do things for themselves and others. They hide their heads in the ground like the proverbial ostrich in the false hope that unseen dangers will go away. Children must not be pushed to face dangers they are unable to cope with, but they do need steady encouragement to overcome those dangers they are capable of overcoming (see Chapter II).

Sometimes well-wishing parents act in a manner that could not possibly produce the expected results. A fourteen-year-old boy was brought to my office by his quite intelligent and concerned parents. "The boy needs psychotherapy," they said. "He is very nervous. He is afraid to swim. He does not play ball with other boys. He avoids them, and plays alone. What will happen to him when he grows up and we can no longer take care of him?"

The boy's own story shed light on his withdrawing behavior. His father's favorite pastime was to ridicule him. "You are a coward," he would say whenever the boy tried to secure some sort of support, "Why won't you swim? It's just water, nothing else! What are you afraid of? Shame on you!"

The father was an athletic, ambitious, and aggressive businessman who was thoroughly disgusted with his son because he did not display physical agility nor aggressiveness. Every summer the family would go to the seashore. The father, who was a good swimmer, would pull his son into the ocean and splash water on him. When the boy had swallowed plenty of ocean water and was almost choking, his father would laugh and push him into deeper water.

Of course, the father did not intend to hurt his son. He just wanted to "help him become a man." He believed that forcing his son to face up to dangers would make him brave. "Then father and son could go to town together! Don't you think so, Doctor?" the father asked.

On one occasion the father pushed the boy into deep water and the boy began to drown. Immediately the father rushed to his rescue and safely pulled him out. He was proud of himself and believed that now that the boy had gone through the worst, he would no longer fear water.

PSYCHOLOGY OF CHILDREN'S FEARS

But the boy was in a state of shock and his fear of water turned into panic. Every summer he developed all kinds of respiratory diseases (of psychosomatic origin) to protect himself from his father's "swimming lessons."

While the boy's mother did not share her husband's enthusiasm for swimming, she agreed with him on several other issues. They both wanted their son to become interested in the family-owned business. The boy was a very good student and excelled in mathematics. "He could become an excellent accountant, for unfortunately he is not aggressive enough to be a lawyer," both parents said.

But the boy, who was ahead of his age group in school, hadn't the slightest interest in business, law, or accounting. He was an excellent student in science and, with the support of a sympathetic teacher, had conducted his own experiments in chemistry.

"Who needs chemistry?" his parents complained. "In a year and a half our son will graduate from high school and go to college. We want him to major in business administration or something similar. He is *our* child, and he should care for his family," they complained, meaning that he should be a carbon copy of his father.

The boy told me about his plans for the future. He wanted to become a chemist, and a great one, but he was unsure of himself. He thought perhaps his father was right, that he was indeed a coward "hiding in a lab from real life." Harsh parental criticism had badly undermined his self-confidence, and he doubted whether he could accomplish anything at all.

He admitted that he did not like football, but had liked baseball and basketball until, unfortunately, his father saw him playing with his peers. He was not the best player, but he was not the worst either. That evening his father entertained some guests by describing, with a lot of humorous gestures, how his clumsy son played ball. This cruel criticism destroyed the boy's desire to play any kind of ball.

This boy's father discouraged his child by forcing him prematurely to face dangers he was unable to cope with. Other parents do not allow their child to cope with any hardships at all and thus perpetuate the child's fears. Some mothers, in particular, believe that by spreading their protective wings about a child they are helping him, when in reality they are stifling him. "You cannot do this," the well-wishing mother says, "let me help you. Mommy will always help you."

A seventeen-year old girl was brought to my office by her mother. The mother complained that her "big daughter" was afraid of "darkness, subways, storms, boys, competition, dogs, you name it." She insisted on being present at the initial interview, and I did not object because I hoped to get some insight into their mother-daughter interaction.

My decision was well rewarded. I suspected that the girl's fears were, if not created by her mother, at least fanned by her attitude. (As will be explained in the following chapters, some fears are innate and common to the entire human race. Parental attitudes and other environmental influences such as relatives, friends, teachers, and schoolmates may help or hinder the child's ability to overcome these fears.)

As the session progressed, I became more and more convinced that the mother's efforts to help her daughter were definitely misdirected. She herself was an outgoing woman, almost flamboyant, and believed that her dynamic personality would set an example for her daughter. Unfortunately, the mother's energy and her impatience prevented her daughter from becoming active on her own

PSYCHOLOGY OF CHILDREN'S FEARS

behalf. All my questions directed to the girl were quickly answered by the mother, who did not allow the girl to say anything on her own.

When subsequently I saw the girl alone, she told me that from early childhood her mother had impressed upon her that she was smarter, brighter, faster, more dependable, more competent, more attractive—in short, a better human being than her daughter. Even at seventeen she was not allowed to do anything on her own. Her mother bought her clothes, combed her hair, supervised her bathing, cut her nails, woke her up in the morning, barred her from the kitchen, and constantly reminded her how much she needed her mother's help. When the girl brought friends home, the mother greeted, treated, and entertained these boys and girls, and later told her daughter with whom she should associate. When the girl went to a party, her mother waited up for her and demanded a detailed report. "This questioning," the girl said, "was really a third-degree interrogation."

The mother firmly believed her attitude was helping her daughter overcome her fears and it took a while before I could convince her otherwise. Months after the beginning of psychotherapy, when the girl dared to buy herself a blouse, her mother called to ask me whether it was appropriate for a seventeen-and-a-half-year-old girl to shop by herself!

Severe states of fear and anxiety may cause regressive phenomena in adults as well as in children. During World War II, I saw panic-driven adults temporarily lose control of their bowels and bladders and regress to baby talk. Severe fears adversely affect insight and foresight, impair judgment and self-control.

Regressive phenomena are even more dangerous in children because they have not had the chance to develop a mature personality structure. The younger the child is, the more damage can be caused to his personality and growth. Battered children who live under the terror of parental wrath and corporal punishment may develop severe emotional disorders.

Anxiety

Though the words "fear" and "anxiety" are often used interchangeably, it is useful to make a clear distinction between them. The physical reactions to fear and anxiety are pretty much the same—they both involve the autonomic nervous system, specifically its sympathetic part, which affects the activity of the gastrointestinal system, increases the secretion of adrenalin, speeds up the heart rate, and so on. However, *fear is an emotional reaction to a specific real or unreal danger,* such as vicious dogs or gobelins, whereas *anxiety denotes a general gloomy feeling of impending doom.*

Fear is a *momentary* reaction to danger. It is based on a low estimate of one's own power as compared to the power of the threatening factor. *A fear disappears with a change in the balance of power.* In the presence of an adult who is perceived by the child as offering protection, the child's fear will be allayed or obliterated. The disappearance of the threatening person, animal, or object will also put an end to the child's fear. And the child's changing estimate of his own power in comparison to the danger will remove his fear.

Anxiety, on the other hand, is *general* and *lasting.* It has a feeling of no specific object but reflects overall weakness, ineptitude, and helplessness. Anxiety is tantamount to the loss of self-esteem and it can paralyze one's life. Expecting an impending doom, one may withdraw from usual activities, become exceedingly tense, irritable, and unproductive. Anxiety may temporarily affect one's intellectual function. The state of anxiety may make a person momentarily forget things he knows, stutter or stammer, and be unable to communicate his thoughts as if his mind has gone blank.

It is important to distinguish between these two emotions in children. Fear is an emotional reaction to a certain threat. The child who fears perceives the threatening person, animal, object, or situation as being *stronger than himself,* and thus capable of *harming him.* Fear is related to perceiving oneself as weak in comparison to the threatening force, but fear can be allayed by the presence of a strong and friendly person, such as a parent, grandparent, or older sibling. It can be also overcome by familiarizing oneself with the source of threat, such as the dark room or a dog.

Anxiety results from an overall feeling of weakness and therefore inability to cope with dangers. A frightened child feels he cannot stand up to a *particular* danger. An anxious child continually underestimates his ability to cope with life in general, or at least with a great many situations. The presence of his mother, familiarity with the dog, does not resolve his uneasiness. Anxiety does not come from without; it comes from within, from the unconscious.

This distinction is especially significant in child psychology. A child who fears dogs may be otherwise a happy child, active and outgoing. His problem is a limited one, and whoever tries to help him can depend on the child's resources. Moreover, the sheer process of growth and development will increase the child's powers and faith in himself, and increased self-confidence may help him overcome his fears.

An anxious child does not have an external problem; the problem is himself and his total personality. He does

CHILDREN'S FEARS

not fear anything in particular, but he feels generally insecure. This insecurity may affect his total behavior, causing learning disabilities, social difficulties, and a variety of problems including some specific fears.

Lucy was a bright ten-year-old girl who was failing most subjects in school, especially mathematics. She was brought for treatment to a psychologist, whom I had been supervising.

Her father, a business executive, could not understand how *his* daughter "could be so stupid." Once in a while he tried to "help" her. He would fire at her one question after another, and demand quick answers. "Multiplication," he said, "is not philosophy. You know it or you do not. Answer fast, one two three, how much is seven times seven, ha?"

The more he tried to "help" her, the more frightened and insecure Lucy became. Because she didn't dare make mistakes, she refused to take chances. Her father called her "dummy," "stupid," "moron," which, of course, did not help. The more "help" he gave her in the form of frequent testing, the more she failed. "What's the matter with our child?" the parents asked.

Lucy was an anxious child. From the day she was born her business executive father and her politically active mother constantly criticized her. Her father wished he had a football-player son (he himself had never been successful in sports), and her mother wished she had a sweet, charming dolly (she thought of herself as rather unattractive). Both parents had done a thorough job of destroying whatever self-confidence Lucy could have mastered, and then wondered why the Good Lord had "punished" them with such an inferior child!

Lucy was quite bright, but she was an anxiety-ridden, frightened child. She was most afraid of being harshly

PSYCHOLOGY OF CHILDREN'S FEARS

criticized, and in school she didn't dare volunteer an answer, even when she knew the subject well. When the teacher asked, "Who was the first President of the U.S.A.?" she knew very well the correct answer, but she wouldn't take chances.

Mathematics was her worst subject, because there it was impossible to hedge. Two and two always equaled four, and one was not allowed to hesitate. She found it safer to withdraw than to venture into an unpredictable world.

As will be explained in detail in Chapter VIII, dealing with children's anxieties differs from dealing with their fears.

Phobia (Displaced Fear)

Sometimes people are so afraid of something that they cannot admit to themselves what they are afraid of. Totally unaware of what frightens them, they may unconsciously develop a fear of something else. This new fear, which displaces the original fear, is usually quite persistent.

A phobia is a constant, compulsive preoccupation with the thing, animal, or person one is afraid of. Consider fear of dogs. A phobic child may be cheerful and happy all the time except when faced with a dog. Then, if very young, he will cry and run to his mother for protection. If older, he will avoid dogs and become tense in their presence.

Sometimes a child is so preoccupied with his fear of dogs that he avoids going to the playground or refuses to play on the street or visit his grandmother or even go to school because he may encounter *some* dog on the way. He may anxiously check the doors and windows at night to make sure no strange dog can break in. The phobia may cause nightmares of dogs chasing him, and the child may refuse to watch a TV show in which a dog appears.

22

CHILDREN'S FEARS

One of my patients, a thirty-year-old married woman, told me of her fear of cats. She maintained that she had always feared cats, and could not recall a time when she did not have "this ridiculous fear."

As our psychotherapy progressed, it became obvious that this was not a genuine fear but a displacement of some deeper fear. She was highly intelligent and knew that kittens could not harm her, but the sight of any cat, big or small, threw her into a panic for reasons beyond her comprehension. Her fear was sometimes quite embarrassing, especially when she had to visit friends who owned cats.

My patient lived with her husband in a two-family house in the suburbs. Both of them worked in Manhattan and went home together even if that meant one of them had to wait for the other. My patient was coming to my office twice a week after work, and her husband often waited for her in my waiting room. Other times she picked him up at his office. It was rare that one of them had to stay in the city so late that the other had to go home alone. Occasionally they went to a show or a restaurant alone or with friends.

One winter day her husband told my patient that he had to attend a meeting that might drag on quite late and my patient decided to go home alone. She left her office as usual at five thirty. It was a cold and windy day in December, and she was eager to get home. This is the story she told me the next day when she came for her psychotherapeutic session.

When she arrived home, she turned on the switch by the stairs leading to their apartment. And hell, what was sitting on the stairs? A big, gray cat. The cat opened his "horrible" bloodshot eyes and closed them again. He did not move. He just sat there on the stairs leading to her

PSYCHOLOGY OF CHILDREN'S FEARS

apartment, motionless, his eyes half closed. Once in a while he opened his eyes.

"A shudder went through my body," my patient confessed, her eyes and voice expressing terror. "I felt cold, very cold. Maybe because the wind was fierce. I trembled. No, it wasn't the wind. It was cold, true, but my entire body trembled. I shook with fear. I tried to be calm and use reason: "I am a big, tall girl, and what could a cat do to me?" I could have chased him away with my umbrella, but I stood there paralyzed, petrified, frozen.

"It occurred to me that I could ring the neighbors' door and wait there for my husband. Luckily, they had a separate entrance on the other side of the house.

"I walked slowly, looking back. I feared that horrible cat would follow and attack me. Isn't it silly, Dr. Wolman, a grown-up woman harboring such a stupid idea?

"The fear was stronger than my reason. Luckily, the street where we live is well lit. I took a few steps, and, oh God, the neighbors' windows were dark!

"It was seven o'clock in the evening. They could not have gone to sleep, so they must be out! They liked to dine out. But if they had gone to a restaurant or to a show, that meant they would not be back before midnight!

"I felt resentment toward my husband. He didn't care! He had let me down in a most trying moment in my life! How could he do this to me! He really didn't give a damn!

"I tried to calm myself. My husband, the poor man, hates business meetings, but this was important and he couldn't have avoided it. I tried to reason with myself. I read some time ago that a neurotic is a person who grew up physically and even intellectually, but part of his personality did not grow up and remained infantile. That's

CHILDREN'S FEARS

me! Stupid me! How can an intelligent adult act so silly!

"Doctor, I was afraid to move away. What would I do if the cat decided to follow me! I had to stand there and keep an eye on him.

"It was getting colder and colder. My feet froze. My knees turned to icicles. I was hungry, tired, miserable, but I could not move, I could not take my eyes off the cat, as if hypnotized by him."

My patient stood on those stairs for five long hours!

Her husband came home at half past eleven to find his wife "half-dead." He raised his voice, the cat ran away, and he took his wife inside.

The entire therapy session was devoted to the previous night's experience. I asked my patient to free-associate, but her unconscious memories were blocked. The word "cat" elicited defensive responses, such as "I told you I hate cats! Maybe I don't hate them, I am just afraid of them! There is nothing I can say about it! I know it's childish but I can't help it! We had no cats in our home! I can't stand their sight! I could vomit at their smell!"

I gave her some signal words: "Bloodshot eyes? Half-closed eyes? What comes to your mind now? Any ideas? Any recollections?"

A shudder went through my patient's body. "My poor mother," she moaned. "She always had eye trouble! Her eyes were often red! She disliked bright light. Quite often she kept her eyes half-closed! *But she was not a cat!!!*

At the next session the patient told me of a dream that made her wake up screaming in the middle of the night. Even in my presence the recollection of that dream gave her a horrible feeling.

"This was a most horrifying dream," she told me, "a real nightmare." She was a little girl, in her parents' home. She had done something wrong. Spilled milk on a new

PSYCHOLOGY OF CHILDREN'S FEARS

carpet or something like that. She was scared, very scared, and she wanted to hide but knew her mother would find her and punish her. She sat in a corner, looking out, and then a big gray cat came along. His eyes were red, blood-shot. They were half-closed. She couldn't take her eyes off the cat. The cat sat quietly for a moment. Then suddenly he leaped and sank his claws in her arm! At this point she woke up screaming with a pain in her left arm.

In the office my patient broke into tears. When she stopped crying, she pulled up the sleeve of her left arm. There were visible scars.

"My mother!" she screamed. "My mother would never forgive anything! She laid in wait and then she attacked! She had long, sharp nails! I was always afraid of her! I could never predict her moods! Sometimes she was nice and cuddly, like a kitten, and then her mood changed and she was vicious and scratched me like a wild cat!"

Obviously my patient could not accept her fear of and hatred toward her dead mother. As a child, she had feared her mother and wished her to die. Quite naturally, she hated herself for hating her mother, especially after her mother died. Her unconscious had displaced the fear and resentment of her mother, and the fear of her own hostile wishes, into a phobia of cats. This phobia was silly on a conscious level but tolerable on an unconscious level, for it was easier and more acceptable to fear and hate cats than to harbor those feelings toward a dead mother.

A few years ago I treated a twenty-year-old man whose main problem was agoraphobia (fear of open spaces). This young man was spending most of his time indoors in his parents' home, refusing to go to work or to college. He didn't dare go out alone, and insisted that a member of his family accompany him on his twice-a-week visits to my office.

CHILDREN'S FEARS

It took a while to unravel the complexity of his fear. He had a violent temper and, unconsciously, harbored aggressive sexual impulses. He feared that he might physically assault girls and rape them, and his fear of his own behavior was transformed (displaced) into a fear of being alone outdoors.

Elation and Depression

Elation and depression reflect, respectively, the positive and negative evolution of oneself. When a person feels strong—that is, believes in his ability to cope with life—he is elated; when he doubts his powers, he may be anxiety ridden and depressed.

Exaggerated self-esteem leads to an irrational manic state. Excessive self-deprecation leads to morbid depression. Alcoholics and drug addicts often experience irrational feelings of power they do not have, and depressive individuals wallow in helpless anger. Maniacs see no danger in dangerous situations, depressives see danger everywhere.

The way a child copes with threats may affect his future emotional development. It is wrong to make a child feel that dangers do not exist and the world is a nursery where a kind mother will take care of all problems. But it is even worse to make a child feel helpless, at the mercy of unsurmountable obstacles and inevitable defeat. A child must be taught to cope with dangers in a rational way and develop a realistic dose of courage.

Courage

Courage is the belief in one's ability to cope with dangers. It is the opposite of fear. Courage is faith in oneself, self-reliance, and self-confidence. It is the feeling that one has enough power to stand up and be counted.

PSYCHOLOGY OF CHILDREN'S FEARS

Brave people have a good deal of self-respect and dignity. True courage is realistic and closely related to a correct estimate of one's own power and the power of the threatening people, animals, or situations. Power without wisdom is plain stupidity, and a person who ignores dangers or confronts them unprepared is not a hero but a brazen fool. Brave men and women think twice before sticking out their necks. They take all the necessary precautions and use all their mental and physical resources in order to overcome the hardships and win. Self-defeating individuals who ignore insurmountable odds and throw themselves into dangerous situations are desperados. They do not display courage but self-destructive despair.

Human life starts in helplessness. Newborns do not have the ability to satisfy their needs (power), and unless someone else who has power (parents or parental substitutes) is willing to take care of and protect them (acceptance), they could not survive. Their fears are alarm bells calling for help from without. Parents should give the child the feeling that he will be taken care of, and at the same time help him grow and mature to the stage where parental help and protection are superfluous. The main parental tasks are to accept the fact that the newborn child is helpless, offer him the necessary security as he is growing, and help him to become a self-reliant individual capable of interrelating with other adults and taking care of his own children.

The degree of courage an individual displays depends on a number of changing factors, and the same individual may act differently in different situations. For one thing, poor health or a run-down physical condition makes one physically weak, and in many (but not all) cases this adversely affects one's courage. Emotional involvement and commitment, self-respect and responsibility, are signs of mental maturity, and also the main ingredients of courage. During World War II, I saw patriotic soldiers courageously and even heroically fulfill their duty. A parent who loves his or her children may reach the highest level of courage in defending them.

Loneliness usually reduces one's courage. The presence of people perceived as strong and friendly—that is, having power and willing to help—greatly enhances one's courage. Most people display more courage in a group action. However, a large crowd can dull one's sense of reality and awareness of dangers, and mob behavior may be more brazen than courageous.

Chapter II.
From Infantile Dependence toward Adult Self-Reliance

There are several reasons why children are less capable than adults of coping with threatening people, animals, and situations. One main reason is lack of power. Children are physically weaker and smaller, less experienced and less wise than adults, and therefore less capable of coping with dangers. And the younger they are, the less power they have, and therefore, the younger they are the more fears they are subject to.

The second reason is their dependence (or acceptance, as defined in Chapter I). Children's need for "allies" is much greater than adults'. Small children cannot survive unless an adult takes care of them and supplies them with food, shelter, and so on. Quite naturally, then, what little children fear most is rejection and abandonment.

In addition to these two main and apparent reasons,

children neither choose the situations they are in nor can they change them. Adults can change their jobs, places of residence, or marital relations, but children are born to and brought up by people they did not choose, and there is not a thing they can do about it.

Adults are also able to create a more or less stable environment for themselves. They can live all their adult years in a certain neighborhood, practice a definite occupation, develop close associations with friends and relatives, and establish a structured daily routine. Children do not have these options. They must move to a new neighborhood and attend a new school whenever their parents decide so, and be forced to face a totally different physical and social environment.

Finally, adults are always adults, and their behavior patterns are more or less circumscribed by sex, age, occupation, religion, and so on. Children's behavioral patterns are continually changing because a child must not remain a child although he is not allowed to be an adult. Growing and maturation are processes of change, and the terms of change are arbitrarily and sometimes whimsically determined by parents.

Since children have very little power of their own, their fears, unless allayed, can play havoc with their mental health. A self-confident person reacts to danger by mobilizing his resources, but a child may be paralyzed by a frightening situation because he has little self-confidence and practically no self-reliance.

Frightened, anxious children often regress to an earlier phase of development where they felt better protected and more secure. A kindergarten-age child may regress to baby talk and a school-age child may become a bedwetter in the face of a threatening situation.

PSYCHOLOGY OF CHILDREN'S FEARS

The Dual Role of Childhood

Several studies have proved that the frequency and severity of a child's fears depend on the child's faith in his or her own forces, such as physical strength, agility, and wisdom, and on the presence of supporting adults. The belief in one's own power is the prime factor in adults— mature individuals *first* count on themselves, and *then* on their friends, relatives, and others—but children must count first on others, on assisting and protecting parents or parental substitutes. Adults' security depends on power first and acceptance second; children's security depends on acceptance by others first and their own power next. Power has been defined as the ability to satisfy needs, and survival is certainly the arch need. Acceptance has been defined as the willingness to satisfy the needs of other people—that is, to help, protect, and defend.

Immature adults tend to believe that somehow somebody will take care of them, protect them, bail them out. They tend to avoid taking rational risks while risking much more by passively waiting for nonexistent saviors.

Children must receive an adequate amount of protection in order to function freely as children. Under no circumstances should children be ridiculed or punished for not being as adult and mature as some parents may wish them to be. A child has the right to be a child, and as such he deserves all the parental protection and acceptance he needs to give him the feeling of security. The very presence of strong and friendly parents or parental substitutes considerably reduces the child's fears.

Children must be guided and helped in the process of reaching maturity. They must be helped to grow stronger and wiser, and develop a realistic estimate of their physical and mental resources.

CHILDREN'S FEARS

They have to be encouraged in the natural process of shifting from dependence on others for their security to self-reliance.

Growth and Maturation

The normal process of maturation and learning does not lead to a complete disappearance of all fears but to the *abandonment of unrealistic fears and the development of realistic fears.* Infants may fear vacuum cleaners, mother's new hairdo, and daddy's new sunglasses, but they do not fear street red lights or the rattling of machine guns. Mature individuals fear red lights and seek cover in war and street fighting; to them, nearby machine-gun fire is more frightening than the heavy barking of distant cannons.

Mentally healthy individuals are realistic, and their perception of things is pretty close to reality. They are capable of distinguishing wish from reality, and whenever they err, they test again and rectify their findings. The picture they have of themselves and others closely corresponds to the truth. They are neither cowardly nor brazen, neither shy nor cocky. *They have the courage to face hardships, and the wisdom to avoid unnecessary risks.*

Children only gradually develop this ability for reality testing. Their innate fears of sharp noises, heights, and so on require *corrective experience.* Children gradually learn and mature, and every child has his own biologically determined speed of maturation and innate ability to learn and profit from experience. Parents should provide the best possible opportunities for growth; they may protect their child from diseases and prevent malformations, but they must be patient, for there is no power in the world that can make a child into a mature adult overnight.

The process of growth is rarely a vertical line. Rather, it is a graph of ups and downs; some fears disappear temporarily and suddenly crop up at a later time. As the

PSYCHOLOGY OF CHILDREN'S FEARS

child's cognitive abilities improve, he may fear things he did not fear before because he was unaware of their potential threat. At the same time, he may become afraid of things he has become familiar with. As his imaginative abilities develop, imaginary creatures and situations may arouse fear.

A child must be helped in this natural process of outgrowing certain fears that appear at a certain age. These fears are normal so long as they come at certain developmental stages, and the child gradually outgrows them. They are abnormal and harmful when they persist and prevent the child from reaching a higher developmental stage.

A child should not be rushed into adulthood, neither should he be infantilized. He should be helped through the necessary steps until he reaches maturity. This means parents must provide understanding and guidance in overcoming infantile, irrational, and imaginary fears, while teaching the child to fear real dangers and to cope with them in rational ways.

Mature men and women experience realistic fears; they are reasonably cautious and do not take unnecessary and silly risks. But they are not afraid to face challenges, to assert themselves, to take calculated risks, and to protect themselves and their dear ones. They are aware of their own power and have the courage to use it.

Individual Differences

There are considerable individual differences in children's susceptibility to fear. No doubt some children are genetically predisposed and show a greater sensitivity than others. Prenatal life and birth may also affect the child's future emotional reactions.

CHILDREN'S FEARS

Not much can be said about heredity besides the fact that there are about eight million possible combinations of genes whenever a male sperm enters a female egg. Brothers and sisters share some physical and mental traits, but it is impossible to predict which traits they will share and to what extent. Small wonder that two children of the same parents can be totally different and react in a radically different manner to the same situation and to parental encouragement or lack of it. Obviously parents need not blame themselves for every unusual sensitivity of their child because a considerable part of the child's personality is determined by genetic, prenatal, and perinatal factors.

Some individual differences must be traced to children's environment and experiences and the way they have been treated by their parents, relatives, neighbors, and teachers. Chapter VIII describes how parents should cope with children's fears; suffice it to say here that every experience and every human personality undergoes changes. Certain experiences and attitudes give the child the opportunity for a better, more healthy development, while adverse conditions and unwholesome attitudes can play havoc with the child's mental health.

The psychological differences between the two sexes illustrate the impact of the environment and its cultural norms. There is no biological evidence that females are cowardly and males brave. In most mammals the males are bigger and stronger, but this does not prove that males are less susceptible to fears. For instance, lionesses are usually more aggressive than lions, and animal mothers display no less courage than the fathers.

In the long history of the human race men have dominated women and ascribed to them the tendency to subservient behavior. For millennia male children have been trained to hide their fears and be self-assertive and brave, while female children have been brought up to be dependent and submissive. Small wonder then that most children's studies in the past pointed to a greater frequency of fears among girls. However, there is no evidence that girls are more susceptible to fears than boys. Every girl and every boy is a distinct personality, and there is no reason to assume that gender is the sole or even a significant factor in susceptibility to fear.

Even in the past some women displayed more courage than most men ever did. The Old Testament tells about the brave woman Judge, Debora, who inspired and led her people in the rebellion against oppressors. Joan of Arc led Frenchmen against the British invaders, and showed more courage than any one of her male compatriots. The British Queen Elizabeth and the Russian Empress Katherine were certainly brave women, and the Israeli Golda Meir and the American Eleanor Roosevelt did not lack courage either.

During the Israeli War of Independence I came across several young men and *women* who, inadequately armed, braved hordes of Arab invaders. I'll never forget the seventeen-year-old Miss B., who joined an active combat unit because her boyfriend had been killed on Mount Castel and, as she told me, "Now I have to fight for two." During World War II many French, Belgian, and Dutch women joined the partisans (Macquis) and fought bravely behind the German lines. Men and women together fought in the Warsaw Ghetto in a tragic defense of human freedom and dignity.

We must finally put to rest the myth of brave men and cowardly women. Courage is not a sex privilege.

Fears and Intelligence

There is a definite relationship between children's fears and the level of their intelligence. Children with superior intelligence are likely to be more aware of real dangers than other children. Bright children have better perception, and usually develop fears early in life. However, the fear of supernatural events is more frequent among less intelligent children.

Undoubtedly the awareness of danger is related to cognitive abilities. Bright children are early aware of dangers, but they are also early in overcoming them. At two or three years of age bright children have more fears than average children, but as the bright children grow older, the relationship reverses, and six-year-old children with superior intelligence have fewer fears than do average children.

Bright children are also less likely to succumb to imaginary fears. They are more inclined to test reality; they learn faster by experience and are more open to persuasion than less bright children.

Fear and Loneliness

Almost ninety years ago the great American psychologist William James wrote, "The great source of terror in infancy is solitude." The absence of a protecting person, parent or parental substitute, is in itself a serious cause of fear, and the presence of such a person mitigates all kinds of fears.

The little child does not have strong muscles, quick legs, bow and arrows, fortresses and bank accounts. Being weak, he fears a lot of things, and as he learns more about life, his fears are likely to increase. Naturally the child grows and gains physical and mental powers and this development eventually will enable him to overcome his fears. But this gradual process requires a continual flow of "safety supplies" from without.

PSYCHOLOGY OF CHILDREN'S FEARS

The fear of abandonment and loneliness may take various forms, but it persists throughout childhood. Children fear loss of their parents by death or divorce; they fear being rejected or sent away from home; they fear being criticized and rebutted; they fear failure in school; they fear punishment for real or unreal transgressions; they fear figments of their imagination. However, *most of all, they fear being alone.*

In the first four or five years of life the physical presence of a protecting parent or parental substitute is the choice method for allaying the child's fears. The availability of the parent the child perceives as *strong* and *friendly* builds the child's feeling of security, makes him less susceptible to fear, and helps him overcome his inevitable developmental fears.

Even the most frightening situations, such as thunderstorms, or strange objects, like a noisy vacuum cleaner or an overdressed relative, become less frightening to a two-year-old if his mother is around and reassures him verbally or by holding his hand. As long as the child feels that he can *trust* his parents and that they will be there whenever he is in danger, he will safely pass through the developmental years and grow toward maturity.

Persisting, Declining, and Growing Fears

Certain fears are typical of the phases of childhood to be described in the following chapters. As the child grows, these fears tend to diminish and eventually disappear. Fears of natural events such as darkness, noise, and storms decline with age, and mature adults rarely fear these natural phenomena. Also fears of imaginary and supernatural dangers such as ghosts, spirits, and goblins disappear in adulthood.

Other fears persist, such as fears of physical dangers, death, sickness, surgery, and bodily injury, of being assaulted by muggers or in war, of car accidents and airplane crashes. While most of these fears persist into adult years, the degree to which they are experienced varies. All people, young and old, fear death, but some are rational and cautious, while others are irrational and allow their fear of death to prevent them from enjoying life.

Also certain fears related to human relations persist all through life, especially the fear of loneliness and isolation. As explained in Chapter I, fear and courage depend on one's estimate of one's power in comparison to the threatening people, animals, or situations. No human being is powerful enough to overcome all dangers, and all human beings derive a great deal of security through association with other people. As mentioned above, children derive their feeling of security mainly from their parents; they *depend* on their parents or other adults.

Anxiety

The child's dependence on adults needs additional explanation. A child cannot fight for survival. He can only seek escape to a more secure place or situation. A frightened infant flees for security to his mother. If he finds security, his fears are allayed. Being sure that he will be protected, trusting his strong and friendly parents, enables him to grow into a self-confident adult.

But if he is not offered protection or if he is unsure that such protection is forthcoming, he may develop an overwhelming anxiety. He may doubt his own ability to cope with dangers. He may feel that he does not deserve to be loved and protected. He may blame himself and others for failing to win them over. Hatred is the Siamese twin of fear, and rejected children hate those who reject them and themselves for being rejected. Severe and persistent states of fear can cause grave damage to the child's mental health and turn him into a panic-driven, self-hating, and/or hate-driven individual.

Chapter III.
The First Year of Life

To be born does not necessarily mean to be ready for life. The human child lives for forty weeks inside the maternal body, enjoying all the privileges of parasitic life. All his needs are taken care of without any effort on his part.

Birth introduces a radical but not a complete change in the situation. The newborn infant must respire on his own, but food and protection are still supplied by the good mother. The newborn child continues to be totally dependent on parental love and care. He has very little if any power of his own and his very survival depends upon parental acceptance.

Small wonder that the infant experiences a variety of fears. Some of the fear reactions are adjustive and useful. They are alarm signals that attract parental attention to potential danger and call for immediate intervention.

Children's fears can be divided into three categories:

(1) fears present at birth, the *innate fears;* (2) fears that appear at a certain age, the *developmental fears;* and (3) fears produced by *traumatic experience.*

Innate Fears

Certain fears are apparently innate, though they do not appear in all children at exactly the same age and in the same manner. The infant's physical and social environment, the way the parents act, and a variety of other factors greatly influence the infant's emotional response. For instance, newborn and very young children react with apparent fright and cry and startle at a sudden loss of support. However, when a loving mother or nurse playfully lets the infant go a few inches up and down, the infant will not necessarily react with crying.

The same applies to loud noises. All newborns and infants are frightened by loud noises, but if they are tightly and affectionately held in mother's arms, and she laughs or smiles, the infant may not be scared.

As a rule, all new and powerful stimuli evoke fear. This fear of the new, the unknown, the unfamiliar undoubtedly has survival value. It is an innate fear common to humans and several animal species. Novel and strange stimuli may signal a potentially dangerous situation, and all living creatures are both curious and suspicious of the new and unknown.

A few-weeks-old infant may be frightened by his mother's new hairdo or father's new dark glasses. A jack-in-the-box must be introduced gradually, and certainly not in the first few months of life. The same applies to quick-moving mechanical toys; parents and relatives may find them amusing but infants do not like them.

Loud and sudden noises elicit fear in most neonates.

CHILDREN'S FEARS

This fear keeps increasing in the first and second year of life, and then begins to decline. It never disappears completely, and even adults may react with a sinking sensation and/or startle at the sudden sharp sound of an explosion. The ability to tolerate continuous, repetitious loud noise also increases with age, but neonate and very young infants should not be exposed to such noises. Should it be impossible to shield them—for example, in a war—parental attitudes can substantially reduce the adverse effect of such exposure.

During World War II, I was in charge of psychological services in one of the Allied nations, and for a while I took care of the mental health of soldiers' families. I visited air raid shelters in cities bombarded by the enemy, and in practically all cases the infants' reaction to nearby explosions depended on their mothers. Whenever the mothers were frightened and hugged the infants, covered their eyes, and so on, most infants had a violent reaction. However, in some air raid shelters we succeeded in developing group morale and close cooperation between the mothers. Whenever there was an explosion, the mothers sang a little strophe, "The daddies beat the bad boy Hitler, bum, bum, bum." There was practically no fear reaction in the infants.

Forcing a child to take risks before he is mentally ready may have an adverse effect and increase his fear rather than decrease it. "What is the matter with you, Johnny, are you chicken? Why can't you go into the dark living room? There are no wild beasts there!" said a well-wishing mother to her "sissy" son, and pushed him gently.

The results were opposite to what the mother had expected. Her child developed sleep disturbances and nightmares, and his fear of dark rooms stayed with him for years.

It is one thing to encourage and another to push.

PSYCHOLOGY OF CHILDREN'S FEARS

Every child is an individual in his own right, and follows his own developmental rhythm. As children grow bigger and stronger, they may dare to do things they never tried before. They certainly should be encouraged and praised for their new achievements, but they should never be forced to do things they are not ready for. Parents must be patient and allow for every child's natural speed of growth and development. As the child grows older, he is tempted to dare and face challenge, but this must be his *own* choice.

Overstimulation

The neonate's ability to absorb oncoming stimuli is limited, so he must not be overstimulated. His fear reaction to loud noises, quickly moving objects, loss of support, and radical changes are defense reactions against potential dangers. Anything new, sudden, powerful, intense, and fast moving presents a threat the newborn is unable to cope with. Overstimulation is harmful for everyone, and the younger and less mature the organism, the greater the danger or potential damage.

The earliest fear reactions to loud sounds, sudden removal of support, and fast-approaching objects are startling, diffuse bodily motions, crying, stiffening of the body, and sometimes fainting. These are not healthy reactions, and the infant should be protected from the frightening stimuli that produce them.

Parents must keep in mind that the younger the child is, the less capable he is of coping with overstimulation and especially with frightening stimuli. The best way to handle these fears is to comfort the child, hold him, make rocking movements, pat him, and talk softly.

Developmental Fears

Quite often, around the twenty-eighth week of life,

CHILDREN'S FEARS

infants develop fears of strangers combined with fear of separation. Parents are sometimes surprised to see their child's changing behavior. The same little cherub who used to smile at everybody and who was pleased to be picked up by anyone who smiled back at him almost over-night becomes negativistic and fearful of strangers, cries in their presence, and holds onto his mother.

This fear of strangers is an almost universal part of the normal process of mental development. The infant has acquired the ability to distinguish between familiar and unfamiliar persons. His perception and span of memory have greatly improved, and he reacts with a pleasurable smile to those who take care of him and supply him with food and affection. Not seeing the familiar faces makes him apprehensive, and the very sight of new and unknown people arouses fear.

Separation anxiety and the resulting fear of annihila-tion are quite pronounced in the second half of the first year of life, usually starting in the seventh or eighth month. Once the infant begins to distinguish between familiar and unfamiliar persons, he becomes more at-tached to those who take care of him. Paradoxically, a one-year-old is more dependent on his mother's presence than a six-month-old, and it is easier to leave the six-month-old with a new babysitter than the one-year-old.

If the mother must be away from the child, she should gradually introduce the babysitter or nurse. It is advisable to have the new person come in for a while and help the mother. This enables the child to get used to the new per-son and gives him the opportunity to perceive her as a friendly.and strong person—that is, willing and capable of taking care of him.

Fear of animals usually starts in the second half of the first year of life. It stems, perhaps, from the combination of three innate fears: fear of sudden motions, of a sudden close approach, and of loud and sudden noises. Dogs certainly fulfill all three conditions: they move fast, they may suddenly come near the infant, and they bark.

There is no need to rush the child in vanquishing this fear. As the parents pet and play with a little dog, the infant may gradually get used to and perceive the dog as a friendly addition to the already familiar household.

Acquired Fears

Some fears originate in traumatic experiences, such as a death in the family or the child's hospitalization and surgery. Certainly parents cannot prevent sad events, but they must spare their child's feelings. If he must be hospitalized, the mother should stay with him in the hospital.

Some minor incidents can elicit fear. For instance, an infant who likes splashing water in a Bathinette or bathtub can suddenly develop fear of both if he slips, or if the water is too hot or he gets soap in his eyes, or for any other reason. Forcing him to go back to the source of his fear will certainly increase that fear. The best course is to wait a while, then gradually reintroduce bathing while reassuring the child and making him trust in maternal protection.

Fear of food at this age is most often fear of feeding. Infants vary greatly in the quality and quantity of food they like, and wise mothers accept their child's whims. After all, the mother herself would not like her appetite and taste to be regulated by someone else.

Overanxious mothers may create unnecessary and sometimes serious problems by forcing the infant to eat food he dislikes, eat more than he likes to, or eat when he has no appetite. The infant may develop fear of one or more kinds of food, gag and throw up, and panic even at a sight of a food he was forced to eat.

CHILDREN'S FEARS

Individual Differences

Startle, crying, "freezing," and clinging to mother are the usual fear reactions of infants. In experiments conducted with four-month-old infants, boys and girls showed no differences in fear reactions. A follow-up study two years later discovered that the boys who were most frightened had less developed speech and poor vocabulary as compared with the boys who were less frightened. The boys who had displayed strong fear reactions at the age of eight months were rather inhibited and apprehensive at the later stage. Nothing of the kind was observed in the girls. Apparently mothers were tolerant of frightened little girls, but they were critical of crying little boys, and their punitive attitude made the boys more apprehensive. Fearful eight-month-old boys were even more fearful at age two and later.

The main symptoms of fear in earliest childhood are trembling, stiffening of the body, crying, and clinging to an adult. Persistent fears may cause loss of appetite, weight loss, nightmares, sleep disturbances, and other symptoms. In the first year of life infants are not able to dismiss fear reaction nor can they easily overcome the resulting tension. It is therefore highly advisable to prevent unnecessary overstimulation and avoid exposure to fear-producing stimuli.

Mental health problems in a way resemble a hammer-and-anvil relationship. A few blows of a hammer may or may not cause damage, depending on the sturdiness of the anvil's surface. The same blows that break a weak surface will cause no damage at all to a very sturdy surface.

It is dubious that all or most mental disorders are caused solely by a traumatic experience. During the Second World War and thereafter I treated several men who had combat exhaustion (also called shell shock), and later I worked with a few former inmates of the Nazi concentration camps. The same or similar shocking experiences did not affect everyone to the same degree. Some people could take more hardship than others, and the differences in their stress tolerance thresholds were usually related to their mental health in early childhood.

As a rule, the older one is, the stronger and better organized he is. Older children are usually better able to take stress and frustration than younger children. In a young child there may be more serious damage to the personality.

It cannot be stressed often enough that a newborn child is physically and mentally helpless. He will have little opportunity for normal mental development unless his early experiences occur in an atmosphere of affection and security. Adverse conditions or lack of love and security in early childhood may cause severe damage to a child's mental health. In my book *Children Without Childhood* I described several cases of severely disturbed children whose personalities were gravely damaged before they had the chance to develop adequate defenses.

The newborn's personality has no defenses. The newborn sleeps or dozes about eighteen hours a day. He wakes up when he is hungry, uncomfortable, or in pain. He cannot take frustration and is helpless in the face of adversities. He needs to feel accepted, loved, and protected. His actions and reactions follow what Freud called *Lustprinzip*, erroneously translated as "pleasure principle" but more accurately the urgency to have needs satisfied immediately. In the earliest phase of life the personality structure is composed of the id, which is a cauldron of instinctual drives that press for an instant discharge of energy. The infant gets panicky when he is hungry and

CHILDREN'S FEARS

food is not forthcoming. He may throw up if the food is not given to him in an atmosphere of tender love and affection. He may develop severe anxiety that will delay his mental development unless he feels loved and protected.

Infants neither speak nor understand the spoken word but they dimly perceive verbal and nonverbal communication. This ability to perceive other people's moods and attitudes (empathy) is common to all infants. A feeding mother who mutters to herself, "Why did I marry this horrible man! And now I am stuck with the baby! Eat, come on, eat, mommy has no time!" her facial expression and tone of her voice will convey hostility the infant is unable to cope with.

As the child grows in a congenial and safe atmosphere, his ego develops and he becomes gradually better prepared to face inevitable frustrations and stresses. The ego is a sort of protective shell and control apparatus that enables the individual to ward off some misfortunes and, what is more important, to control his id impulses and avoid unnecessary troubles.

In short, the same blows of a hammer can break a glass surface but will barely dent wrought iron. Infants must be adequately protected so they can grow stronger and become prepared to cope with inevitable frustrations and stresses.

Chapter IV.
The Toddler

The Yes and No Age

The second year of life brings significant changes in the child's life. This is the time the child is weaned from nipples and learns to walk and talk and explore new experiences and things. As the toddler begins to enjoy his new powers, his parents must set limits on his behavior, including his hitherto free bowel and bladder movements. The second and third year of life are full of discovery and adventure, such as pulling the tablecloth, spilling milk, and playing with food, but at the same time the child must cope with mother's unheard of and totally unexpected demands concerning his bowel movements and urination.

Toilet training can become a traumatic experience for both mother and child unless it is properly handled. Certain negative personality traits and anxiety states develop at this *anal stage* of development. Usually in the second or third year of life toddlers derive considerable pleasure from excretion, and learn to increase this pleasure by delaying emptying their bowels, with concomitant stimulation of the mucous membranes of the rectum.

In his *Standard Edition of the Complete Psychological Works* (Vol. 16, p. 315) Freud states:

> Infants experience pleasure in the evacuation of urine and the content of bowels, and they very soon endeavor to contrive these actions so that the accompanying excitation of the membranes in these erotogenic zones may secure them the maximum possible gratification. . . . The outer world steps in as a hindrance at this point, as a hostile force opposed to the child's desire for pleasure. . . . He is not to pass his excretions whenever he likes but at times appointed by other people. . . . In this way he is first required to exchange pleasure for value in the eyes of others.

According to Freud, the infant sees in his feces part of his own body and is unwilling to part with them. He usually offers resistance to maternal demands, and may try to exercise sole control over his movements. Many infants act aggressively in elimination, thus combining libido and hate in anal eroticism by the sadistic holding and expelling of feces. Resistance against bowel training is an expression of rebellion against adults.

The anal stage appears to be ridden with another ambivalence besides expulsion-retention. Masculinity and femininity should be distinguished at this stage by activity and passivity, respectively. Masculine impulses, such as scoptophilia (gazing), onlooking, curiosity, and the desire to manipulate and to master, may develop into cruelty and sadism. Feminine impulses, on the other hand, usually represent a passive desire connected with the anal and the feminine erotogenic zones. The rectum can be easily stimulated by accepting a foreign body that enters it. This

PSYCHOLOGY OF CHILDREN'S FEARS

anal ambivalence of masculine-active expulsion and feminine-passive reception of a foreign body may lead to a confusion of sexual roles in adulthood.

Abraham, in *Selected Papers*, p. 433, has suggested a subdivision of the anal stage into the anal-expulsive and the anal-retentive stages. In the earlier, expulsive phase the infant enjoys the sadistic pleasure of expulsion. Folklore and slang bear witness to these anal-aggressive tendencies, as preserved in the scatological language used by adolescents and some adults. At the later, anal-retentive stage the infant may develop affection for feces. Feces, after all, are the first possession the infant may give to his beloved mother, and as such they are the prototype of a gift and later of gold and money. In dreams feces may symbolize babies, since children often believe that childbirth is a process similar to elimination. Also, children often consider the penis as being analogous to the column of feces that fills the mucous tube of the bowel.

The anal-retentive phase is usually considered to be the source of tenderness, defined as the wish to preserve and take care of. Freud accepted Abraham's suggestions on this point and elaborated on the concept of tenderness as distinguished from the anal type of love. Even though tenderness seems to originate in the wish to keep and preserve feces, gradually the care spreads to all pleasurable objects and grows into a consideration for the mother, whom the infant wishes to keep and preserve as a future source of gratification. Abraham maintained that the "retention pleasure" outweighed the "elimination pleasure." As tenderness spreads, the child begins to care for his property and pets, handling them carefully and with tenderness.

The particular method of toilet training used by the mother and her feelings concerning defecation may have far-reaching effects upon the formation of specific traits and values in the child. If the mother is very strict and repressive in her methods, for example, the child may hold back his feces and become constipated. If this mode of reacting generalizes to other ways of behaving, the child may develop what is known as a retentive character, becoming obstinate and stingy. Another child, presented with the same repressive measures, may vent his rage by expelling his feces at the most inappropriate times. This is usually considered the prototype for all kinds of expulsive traits, such as cruelty, wanton destructiveness, temper tantrums, and messy disorderliness. If, on the other hand, the mother pleads with her child to have a bowel movement and praises him extravagantly when he does, the child usually acquires the notion that the whole activity of producing feces is extremely important.

A matter-of-fact approach is the rational one to toilet training. The mother should follow the natural biological rhythm of *her* child. She should not start toilet training before her child is ready, notwithstanding the horrendous fact that the neighbor's child who is a full six months younger is already toilet trained while her own child is still soiling his diapers.

Some children mature faster than others, but a slow pace does not necessarily mean a child is a mental retard. Many gifted individuals develop slowly but ultimately reach a much higher level than fast developers. Speed is not a crucial factor in child development, and children must not be rushed. This stricture against applying arbitrary rules holds for all aspects of the child's life, be it walking, talking, control of bowels and bladder, or practically everything else.

A wise mother is aware that undue rush may frighten a child who is not ready to do the things she may wish him

PSYCHOLOGY OF CHILDREN'S FEARS

to do. She must watch her child's behavior and use her judgment—is he ready for the new function or not? There is nothing wrong in trying to start a child on a new activity, provided the mother does not expect instant success or resent the child for failing. Walking and toilet training must not be pursued with an iron hand. The mother should give her child a chance to do what she wants him to do. If he is successful, she should praise him, but realize that initial success does not guarantee continuous success. Learning is a trial-and-error process, and no one has ever learned to type or to play piano on the first trial, and certainly not to keep balance in walking nor to control the bowels.

When the mother notices that the infant moves his bowels every day at more or less the same time, she may put him on a pot or on a special toilet seat.

Infants are curious and they wonder what is coming out of their anus. They may like to play with, to touch, or to smear their feces. This they cannot be allowed to do, but threats and punishments may cause serious fears and anxiety states.

The flushing of the toilet and the disappearance of the feces may give rise to a fear of annihilation (see Section 7) since toddlers view their feces as part of their body and may fear that they too will be flushed away. In most cases maternal reassurance will suffice, but there is no reason to force a frightened child to sit on an adult toilet seat when a portable pot can just as well serve for his toilet training.

A repressive and punitive maternal attitude can turn toilet training into a senseless power contest. The frightened child holds onto his feces for dear life and gradually develops retentive, obstinate, and frugal traits. The desperate mother becomes even more irritable and more punitive, until the scared child may fear to eliminate.

CHILDREN'S FEARS

Some children cannot fall asleep because they fear they will lose control of their bowels.

Rational mothers do not expect quick results. A toddler can, for a while, be a "model child" and move his bowels when expected. Suddenly the model child will regress and soil himself in a most unpredictable way. The mother should take this regression calmly and understand that the process of maturation is one of ups and downs. She should not react to failures, but encourage and praise success. A toddler who grows in an approving and congenial atmosphere without threats and fears of punishment will learn adequate self-control.

Toddlers are not angels, and unless parents act in a firm but affectionate and understanding manner, this stage will be full of unnecessary conflicts, fears, and anxieties. Punishing a child because he is unable to live up to their expectations will greatly contribute to his fears and feeling of inadequacy. Parents must keep in mind that statistical averages look neat on paper, but every child has his own developmental speed.

Apparently the toddler wants to have cake and eat it, too. He is willing to bravely venture into the kitchen cabinets provided his protecting mother is there. He is daring as long as he is sure of parental presence, protection, and approval. The minute he loses sight of his mother, all his courage is gone.

Most fears in the first year of life are innate, and some of them continue for several years. Fears of sudden loud noises, of strangers, of change and separation do not disappear in the second and third year of life. To the contrary, some of these fears become more frequent, for in the second and third year of life, as the child's cognitive abilities improve and expand, the child learns by *imitating adults* and by his *own experience*.

PSYCHOLOGY OF CHILDREN'S FEARS

Fear of *strangers,* of *change,* and of *separation* are the most frequent fears at this age.

Separation Fear

In the second and third year of life fear of separation is probably the worst of all. The infant develops a profound attachment to *his* mommy, *his* daddy, *his* home, bed, and chair, and insists on continuity and sameness. This is probably the most conservative age, for the most daring toddler feels secure only if he can hold onto what he already knows.

If a mother must go to work, she should gradually introduce the babysitter, relative, or nurse, and let her come to the house while she is still at home in order to give the infant a chance to familiarize himself with the new person.

At this age hospitalization can be a shocking experience, for it represents the three worst things: separation, change of environment, and threat of physical pain. It is therefore advisable that the mother stay in the hospital with the sick child and bring from home his favorite teddy bear and other toys. Pain may be unavoidable, but the mother's presence and calm reassurance will mollify its impact. An overanxious mother may unwittingly increase her child's fears, and her overprotective behavior may throw the child into a panic.

Fear of Annihilation

The fear of annihilation appears in the second or third year of life as the infant's perceptual abilities improve and he is capable of noting that things do disappear.

When the water in the bath disappears, many a toddler fears he too will go down the drain. The disappearance of feces in the toilet bowl may give rise to a fear that he too will be washed away with the feces.

The fear of annihilation, as irrational as it is, is actually fear of death. It must not be ridiculed or frowned at. The infant does not need scientific explanations but a hug and a kiss and a few reassuring words (see Section 7).

Fear of Going to Sleep

The fear of sleep has a variety of causes. Separation fear and the fear of soiling and bedwetting are probably the most frequent.

Criticism and punishment will increase the toddler's fears. He may fear being rejected, abandoned, or given away to strangers. He may resent his angry parents and fear his own resentment.

These fears will not last too long if parents are patient and reassuring and stay home until the child is asleep. A favorite toy or a security blanket may assuage the child's fear.

Fear of Animals and Engines

Toddlers tend to believe that pet animals, toys, and inanimate objects have the same thoughts and feelings as human beings. A dog or a cat may be suspected of liking or disliking him, the teddy bear or the doll of feeling cold at night, the toys of feeling lonely and crying because they want to sleep in his little bed. The worst enemy is the loud, noisy, and mean vacuum cleaner. He does not like to be locked in a closet, and when he is taken out, he is furious.

All these and other fears described in Part Two of this book require parental understanding and protectiveness but not overprotectiveness.

Handling Toddlers' Fears

There are two main methods of how *not* to handle a

PSYCHOLOGY OF CHILDREN'S FEARS

toddler's fears. These are punishment at one extreme and overprotectiveness at the other. The obstinate ingenuity of a toddler can drive the most sensible mother up the wall. At bedtime the child who fears going to sleep (he suspects his parents will go out as soon as he closes his eyes) will every few minutes need to go to the bathroom or suddenly require one more sip of milk. There is nothing wrong in setting limits in a calm, firm, and friendly voice. The parents' self-assuredness makes the child feel more secure, but their anger makes him more scared and upset.

Parental impatience, irritation, or anger are often perceived by the child as outright rejection. At this age the child cannot help feeling scared and lonely, even when his parents are in another room. The fear of abandonment motivates him to things that annoy his parents, but what he is asking for is to be reassured that they will not leave him alone.

To get angry at a scared child is tantamount to punishing him for being insecure and overdependent. Punishment certainly does not make him more secure and more independent. It will make him more unhappy and more insecure, and certainly more dependent. Children who receive plenty of love and reassurance are better prepared to strike out on their own. A child who feels accepted and secure does not mind being left for a few hours in a nursery or kindergarten, but an insecure child clings to his mother's apron (see Chapter V). In other words, the more assurance the infant receives, the less he will need it later in life. Children who feel insecure may need protection for years and years.

The second worst method is overprotection. A child needs *strong* and friendly parents (see Chapters I and II). Weak, undecided, worrisome parents undermine the toddler's feeling of security. So does overprotectiveness. Toddlers are not easy to handle, and an annoyed mother may feel guilty for resenting the child and then try to compensate by overprotection. Needless to say, overprotection increases the child's fears, for if mother worries so much, things must be bad indeed.

Toilet training must not be accomplished at the price of unnecessary anxiety in the child. If a child refuses to go to sleep because he fears he may soil or wet his bed, he should be reassured that he is doing fine and a little failure here and there does not matter.

Some childhood fears are rational and contribute to future adjustment. Any fear of a real danger is useful and should be reasonably encouraged. As the child grows and learns more about his environment, the range of his fears widens.

Certainly not all fears are useful and help adjustment. Some childhood fears, especially fears of imaginary creatures, are useless and even harmful. Some fears outlive their usefulness; they are justified in early childhood but become useless and regressive in later years. Parents are gardeners; they watch children grow and supply them with all the care and love necessary for a normal growth.

(More about parents in Chapter VIII).

Chapter V.
Preschool Years

New Experiences

Children's fears come and go, but almost 90 percent of children develop certain fears appropriate for their age. Three-, four-, and five-year-old children have a rich fantasy life that causes them to fear imaginary creatures. They are also able to project their feelings on others, identify themselves with whatever they see, and experience several new fears.

Some of these fears are rational. Naturally, parents caution children against putting their fingers in electric outlets, leaning out of windows in high-rise buildings, playing with sharp knives and matches, picking up broken glass, and so on. They warn children not to tease dogs, not to catch bees, and not to get too near a hot stove. They do not allow children to follow strangers on the street or in the playground or to cross the street on the red light. All

CHILDREN'S FEARS

these warnings are intended to make the child aware of real dangers.

Children at this age are anything but realistic, and they often fear unreal dangers while paying little attention to real ones. Many children do not heed parental guidance and venture into harmful situations. At the same time they tend to develop their own collection of not too rational fears.

Preschool children have lots of fears. They fear dark rooms, strange noises, fire engines, strange people, doctors, hospitals, animals (especially large dogs and snakes), their own dreams, ridicule, magic, injuries, getting hurt, their own death, goblins, spooks, bogeymen, scary stories, scary movies, and a multitude of objects (e.g. vacuum cleaners) that could do no possible harm to them.

Declining and Growing Fears

From the age of two to six years there is a gradual decline in certain fears while new fears appear. The fear of being left alone, for instance, seems to be greatest in the fourth year of life and usually declines in the sixth year.

The majority of children this age fear dark rooms. This fear reaches its peak in the fourth year, drops somewhat in the fifth year, and in most cases disappears in the sixth year.

Fear of strangers is very high in the second and third year of life and slowly goes down in the fourth and fifth year. Most children do not fear strangers in their sixth year. They have become more selective and can distinguish a nice person from a bad one. Increased exposure to other children and adults helps to reduce this fear.

Fear of snakes increases with age; it is highest in the fourth year, but it may persist much longer.

PSYCHOLOGY OF CHILDREN'S FEARS

The fear of large dogs is at its peak in the third year of life, and it may last for two or three years.

Fear of Separation

Separation fear is one of the most common fears at this age. Now the child knows on whom he depends, and develops a strong attachment to his parents, grandparents, or other family members and parental substitutes.

At this age children are possessive and jealous. A child may demand the entire attention of his (or her) mother, nurse, or babysitter, and insist that the mother's hand, which belongs to him, should not caress or carry another infant, sibling, or anyone else. When friends or relatives drop in, the child may sulk if *his* mommy or daddy kisses the intruder.

Possessiveness is a perfectly normal psychological trait and need not be discouraged. People who care for nothing and feel nothing belongs to them are psychological drifters. Possessiveness plays a highly important role in normal child development. As the infant discovers his own body, he tremendously enjoys his discoveries. "That's me, little Michael or little Martha. That's *my* hand, my nose, my toes." This awareness of oneself is a core concept in the child's *body-image* and *ego* development, and is a healthy sign.

It is highly important to give the child an opportunity to accumulate his own little possessions and to develop attachment to "his" cupboard, chair, bed, and a corner of his own. Let him take care of his little possessions, for the more he feels in charge of things that belong to him, the more secure he feels. A security blanket and a favorite teddy bear are part of normal development.

It is irrational to expect a child at this age to cherish

socialistic ideals of common property. A child must establish himself first before he can become capable of sharing and giving. His selfish possessiveness is hardly abnormal, for even well-adjusted adults are not always willing to share their possessions.

As the child grows and develops emotional attachments to parents, relatives, neighbors, and peers, he himself will occasionally volunteer limited sharing and giving. He may offer a piece of candy to his mother or playmate, especially if he has profited by their generosity and feels loved and secure in their presence.

Love is possessive, and those who love do not want to share or to part with their loved ones. Husbands and wives who practice "swapping" do not care for each other. Such casual bonds do not last too long. Open marriages are the first step to broken marriages, for those who love are not too eager to renounce their bonds.

Normally children become attached to their parents, relatives, and friends, and don't want to share them. Wise parents do not criticize possessiveness, but find a way to reassure the sensitive child that they will never abandon him, thus indirectly helping him to conquer his fear of loss when they express affection for other people.

Insecurity breeds excessive jealousy. A secure child feels that his parents will never leave him and therefore does not perceive their attention to other people as a threat. A worried child needs encouragement, such as a father who says "I love you very much, and there is nothing wrong if I kiss someone else. I love you very, very, very much, because *you* are *my* nice little boy." *My, you*—the possessive and personal pronouns—emphasize belongingness and alleviate fears of abandonment (see Section 3).

PSYCHOLOGY OF CHILDREN'S FEARS

Fears of Animals and Objects

At this age many children develop a fear of animals, especially big dogs. There is no reason to ridicule a frightened child or force him to approach a growling German shepherd. It is best to introduce the child to little puppies and enable him, at his own speed, to play with bigger dogs and gradually gain more courage.

When a child fears dark rooms, he fears both the unknown and loneliness. Forcing him to enter a dark room will only increase his fears. A wise parent turns on the light, holds the frightened child's hand, walks with him into the room, and points to familiar objects.

A child who fears the ocean could be gradually encouraged by wading in shallow waters in a swimming pool. A child who fears a vacuum cleaner should be shown a nonactive one, its parts, and mechanism. Knowledge and familiarity reduce fears.

Parental Influence

Some children's fears stem from imitating their parents. Studies have shown that when mothers fear thunderstorms, insects, or dentists, their children will likely develop the same fears. Parent-induced fears are usually long-lasting (sometimes well into adulthood), for it is quite difficult to rid oneself of a fear that is constantly exhibited by one's parents. These are frequently the most exaggerated, for if a powerful parent fears dentists, what can a little child do?

I once had a lady in psychoanalytic psychotherapy who panicked whenever she saw people drinking coffee, and would not allow her husband and children to drink coffee in her presence. After a while it was discovered that her mother feared coffee and believed that it prevented growth and caused shrinking of bones and muscles.

Sexual Fears

Some fears at this age are related to sexuality. Almost every four- or five-year-old boy desires to possess his mother physically, the notion of which he has derived from his observations or from intuitive surmises of sexual life. He may try to seduce her by showing her the male organ of which he is the proud owner. The boy tries to take his father's place, for though he loves and admires his father, at the same time he views him as a competitor and wishes to get rid of him.

At this phase the penis becomes the main source of pleasurable sensations. In addition to the desire to be fondled, a definite need emerges for active pursuit and thrust with the penis.

The little boy is aware of his inferiority in comparison to his father, whose penis is larger. He is afraid that his father will punish him for masturbation, and for desiring the mother. If the boy has had a chance to notice the difference between male and female organs, the castration threat becomes very real and shocking. He may believe that all people originally have a penis but that it is sometimes cut off by an omnipotent father. Castration fear is much stronger than the (oral) fear of being eaten or the (anal) fear of losing body content.

The fear of castration forces the boy to abandon his incestuous desire for his mother. Some boys give up masturbation altogether and develop a passive attitude similar to that of the mother. This passive attitude conceals an increased fear and hatred of the father. Resentment toward the father often develops into a defiant attitude toward all men in authority. Affection for the mother often

PSYCHOLOGY OF CHILDREN'S FEARS

turns into a dependence relationship, into a passive need to be loved. Overattachment to the mother, to feminine components, and partial identification with the mother may lead to a submissive attitude toward women in the future.

In my psychotherapeutic practice I have come across several cases of sexual dysfunction in males related to their childhood conflicts. Normally boys resolve their infantile sexual conflict by identification with the father and acceptance of the male sexual role. In school years (called by Freud "the latency period") boys associate with boys and avoid girls. The presence of a friendly and forceful father helps them in this process of psychosexual identification.

In some instances the apparent weakness of the father, or his absenteeism or lack of interest in his son, prevents the normal process of psychosexual (gender) identification and creates a variety of sexual maladjustments in the child.

One of my patients, a thirty-year-old man, could not sustain an erection and could not have normal sexual intercourse. Impotence brought him to my office.

Soon his dreams revealed the underlying infantile sexual conflicts. He dreamed that a king was about to leave his country, and everyone seemed to be very sad. Apparently, the king was never to come back. The queen stood alone on the seashore, crying. Suddenly, the eyes of everyone turned in the dreamer's direction, as if expecting from him to take care of the queen. The dreamer woke up frightened.

The meaning of the dream was partly transparent. The dream reactivated his infantile oedipal wish to get rid of the father and possess the mother—and the fear of having this incestuous wish come true woke him up.

His fear of women was actually a fear of committing incest and being punished for it. He had always put women on a pedestal, as if any girl he met were his mother, and the unconscious thought of committing incest caused loss of erection.

My patient also had recurrent and frightening castration dreams. Any time his dreams included sexual arousal, something terrible happened. Either his leg was cut off, his head chopped off, or he suffered some other horrible injury.

In some cases, when the mother is strong and aggressive and the father is weak, the little boy represses his phallic strivings toward his mother. Instead of trying to possess her, he identifies with her and forms a passive affection for his father. This *negative* Oedipus complex may lead to homosexuality.

Sexual fears need not be hushed-hushed. Parents can explain to their male or female child that these are usual fears and will soon disappear.

In most cases firm and reassuring parents enable the little boy to identify with his father and the little girl to identify with her mother. Identification with the parent of the same sex greatly helps in resolving infantile sexual fears. The full resolution of sexual fears should take place in adolescence, when boys become girl-crazy and girls boy-crazy, and move toward a mature choice of their life partner (see Chapter VII). Parents need not hesitate to talk about sex, but should remember that actions speak louder than words. Their mutual affection and rational attitude toward their children will allay the children's fears and guide them toward maturity. In extreme cases of sexual fear professional help may be needed.

A child who frequently masturbates may develop all kinds of horrible fantasies. This child needs reassurance and, probably, a more active life.

Fear of Death

The fear of death is universal, but most people do not

PSYCHOLOGY OF CHILDREN'S FEARS

think of it unless someone close to them dies or they themselves are sick, wounded, in a dangerous situation, perturbed, or depressed. A child of three, four, or five years rarely thinks of death unless he or she is anxious, or feels unloved and rejected.

Some children who do feel loved and secure still develop a fear of death. When someone in the family dies, they may identify with the deceased person and wonder whether this could happen to them also. In times of emergency, riots, and war children's fears of death substantially increase.

The best way to handle this fear is to reassure the child and make him or her feel secure, active, and happy. Death is inevitable, but active and happy children rarely think of it.

Fear of One's Own Hostility

At this age many a child overrates his own power. Some children even believe that their words will cause things to happen.

This belief in their own magic power may play havoc with the child's feeling of security. A child who says in anger to a parent, "Drop dead," may fear that his words will kill the parent and develop a frightening guilt feeling and fear of severe punishment.

Some children go even further and fear not only words but also unexpressed feelings and thoughts. They fear that their hostile attitude toward a punishing parent may cause that parent harm. Should the parent get ill or suffer an accident, the child may blame himself.

The most effective reassurance is to explain to the child that everybody gets angry occasionally, but this does not mean anything, and nobody ever got hurt because somebody disliked him.

CHILDREN'S FEARS

Imaginary Fears

Preschool children are very curious. They shower their parents with innumerable questions—"What is this?" "Why is it so?" Being self-centered, they seek connections between what is going on and their own life and often arrive at far-reaching and totally illogical conclusions.

Preschool children are capable of imagining non-existing things and situations, and ascribe human intentions to animals and even inanimate nature. Sometimes the fear of goblins and spooks represents the child's fear of his own hostile feelings.

Children of three to six are unable to clearly and consistently distinguish make-believe from reality. They may fear figments of their own imagination, and it is not advisable to add to their fears. Parental warnings and punishments, if necessary, should be succinct and directed to the child's level of understanding, such as short-term deprivation of some toy, little pleasure, or the like. Scaring the child with policemen, bogeymen, or kidnappers is exceedingly harmful because this is a veiled threat of abandonment, which is the worst thing that can happen to a child. Moreover, this kind of threat fans morbid imagination and drives the child into a state of continuous and unhealthy panic.

Children at this age are sensitive and their minds must be spared. Frightening stories can adversely affect their mental health, and scary movies and TV programs may cause severe damage. Mighty mice, monsters, gangsters, and witches may amuse TV producers and some other immature adults, but they play havoc with the child's mental health (see Section 53).

Communication and Fears

Children who act out their fear on the first day of

PSYCHOLOGY OF CHILDREN'S FEARS

nursery school or kindergarten are not necessarily maladjusted. Some children who do not cry and cling to their mother are more frightened than those who do. The initial expression of fear does not necessarily indicate future difficulties, and the frequent expression of fear does not necessarily prove the child is particularly fearful. Usually, as the child grows older, his overt expression of fear declines. A toddler startles, screams, cries, and flees, but the preschool child preoccupied with fear of imaginary objects does not scream nor can he flee from figments of his own imagination.

Parents should encourage children to communicate their fears. Just talking about fears alleviates them and makes them less threatening. It prevents the feeling that one is alone with his fears and worries. It also improves the parent-child relationship, and proves that the child can trust his parents. A hidden fear can give rise to displacement (phobia) and anxiety, while an expressed fear will enable the parents to offer rational explanation and encouragement.

Chapter VI.
Middle Childhood

In middle childhood (six to eleven) there is some decline in fears related to bodily safety. Children fear sickness, injury, and germs less, and are somewhat less afraid of doctors and dentists. There is also a decline in the fear of dogs, noises, darkness, and storms, and an increased ability to accept temporary separation. There is no significant decline in fears of supernatural forces such as ghosts, witches, and so on.

Most of the new fears are related to school and family. Fears of ridicule by parents, teachers, and peers, as well as of parental disapproval and rejection, increase at this age. The latter may be a contributory factor to school phobia (see Section 52). Fear of failing in school, fear of teachers and bullies come to the fore.

PSYCHOLOGY OF CHILDREN'S FEARS

Worry about Parents

Many children this age become concerned with their parents' health, financial success, interaction with relatives and neighbors, and their social status. These worries may be considerably aggravated by parental behavior. Parents who present themselves to their children as worrisome, weak, helpless creatures greatly contribute to their children's fears.

It is quite natural for school-age children to become aware of their family's problems and worry about their parents. So long as parents do not impose their anxieties and worries on the children, the children's fears will remain within normal limits. Unfortunately, some parents overcommunicate with their children, or tell each other things they should not say in the presence of a child. The father's loss of a job may not necessarily be a catastrophe, but if communicated in a manner that implies immediate starvation, it will seem to be one. Parents who occasionally disagree and exchange harsh words in front of a child may leave him terrified and expecting violence and divorce.

Some parents, wittingly or unwittingly, make their child feel guilty for *their* true or imaginary misfortunes. A sensitive eight- or nine-year-old may come to believe it is his fault his father did not get an expected raise or suffered business losses. Guilt feelings may give rise to a disturbing state of anxiety that interferes with the normal process of child development (see Section 23).

Fears of physical danger, such as being hurt, poisoned, kidnapped, or having to undergo surgery, are quite common. These fears will persist into adulthood, and they have survival value. Often they are related to the fear of being abandoned by parents through the death of one of them, divorce, or some other reason. These fears are typical of normal childhood.

Fear of Parents

Overdemanding and hypercritical parents elicit resentment. A child who fears criticism for being unable to meet the high standards set by his parents perceives his parents as strong and hostile. He may harbor hostile feelings toward them to the point of wishing them dead. These hostile feelings make the child feel guilty and increase his misery. Many children this age believe in the magic power of thoughts and words. They may fear their hostile wishes will come true and they thus develop unconscious conflicts, anxieties, and phobias.

When the parents are unfriendly, impatient, easily irritated, and punitive, the child may develop a frightening fantasy that he or she is adopted.

No child can safely take parental rejection. A school-age child takes temporary separation well and can spend a pleasant day at a grandmother's house or an uncle's farm or in a summer camp. This greatly depends upon his trusting his parents. As long as he is sure they love him and will pick him up when they promised to, he can spend cheerful days away from home.

Sleep-away Camp

The first day in a sleep-away summer camp may produce a good deal of fear and anxiety. The little boy or girl away from home for the first time may experience separation anxiety and fear of the unknown. The child may cry, have no appetite, develop nausea and diarrhea, high urinary frequency, and insomnia. These symptoms indicate he was probably not ready for a sleep-away camp.

The best sign of readiness is enthusiasm. When a

PSYCHOLOGY OF CHILDREN'S FEARS

child's best friends are going to camp and he wants to be with them, when he asks to be sent to camp, he is ready for a prolonged separation from his parents.

Getting Lost

One of the most frightening things that can happen to an anxious child is to get lost. This may happen when he goes out with his mother and she stops on the street or in a park to chat with her friends, or he may become separated from her in a crowded department store.

The physiological symptoms of this type of fear of abandonment and loneliness are quite apparent. The child cries and perspires; his pulse and respiration rate are significantly increased; he has no appetite and refuses to take food offered by friendly strangers; he may develop nausea and diarrhea, and even vomit and lose bowel and bladder control.

Irrational Fears

Rational fears are related to truly dangerous things: big dogs, snakes, serious injury, surgery, loss of parents, or loss of their love. However, many children are possessed by fear of supernatural beings, omnipotent burglars and kidnappers, bogeymen, and other imaginary creatures.

Irrational fears are not a calamity nor do they prove that little Mary or Jimmy is losing his or her mind and needs instant professional help. To the contrary, these fears prove that the child is capable of imagining things and his intellectual abilities are expanding.

There is, however, a highly important rule that must be strictly followed. The name of the rule is *reality testing.* *Parents must help the child draw a clear-cut line between make-believe, storytelling, and fantasy on the one hand, and reality on the other. Whenever the child talks about witches, spooks, and*

Mighty Mouse, or other characters he has read about, seen on TV, or invented himself, parents should neither ridicule him nor join him in his fantasy world. They should instead remind him that this is just make-believe, and everybody can tell tall tales.

Imagination is necessary to a child's normal development but it must be treated carefully. Unnecessary fanning of the imagination is unhealthy. Scary TV programs that give the impression of being real happenings elicit morbid fears and may adversely affect the child's mental health.

School

Many psychologists have studied the reaction of six-to-eleven-year olds to test situations in school. Anxious children perform worse when watched by parents or teachers.

If a child complains that a teacher dislikes him or is unfair to him, parents should not immediately take sides for or against the teacher but, if the situation is serious, meet the teacher and try to solve the problem in a friendly manner. Blaming the child will increase his feelings of loneliness and rejection; blaming the teacher may create more conflict. As a rule, a conference with the teacher and the school guidance counselor will put an end to whatever misunderstanding existed.

It may be more difficult to handle a child's fears of a classroom bully or a hostile clique of peers. In most situations the child should be encouraged to stand up for and defend himself, but sometimes parents must solicit the intervention of the school psychologist or guidance counselor to clear it up.

Problems of Communication

Children at this age are often inclined to hide their fears to avoid being ridiculed and labeled "baby" or

PSYCHOLOGY OF CHILDREN'S FEARS

"chicken." Suffering in silence can be misinterpreted as a sign of maturity.

Hiding fears does not put an end to them so the child who is afraid to communicate his fears sometimes develops displaced fears (phobias) or a deep-rooted feeling of inadequacy and helplessness. Parents should therefore keep the channels of communication open and encourage their child to share his feelings and experiences with them. This does not imply parental overprotectiveness; just showing the child that he is listened to and understood will give him courage in facing dangers and hardships.

There is no one standard way of dealing with a silent fear. A lot depends on the personalities of the parents and their children, and there are no foolproof prescriptions for making a child express his fears.

Love alone is not enough; taking care of children requires a lot of common sense and understanding. Usually parents know when a child is worrisome and upset. Sometimes he does not eat well, or has difficulties falling asleep, or is reluctant to go to school. A child who fears parental criticism will naturally hide his fears and anxieties; why add insult to injury?

If the congenial atmosphere at home facilitates wholesome communication, if parents converse with their child in a friendly manner, if they admit that it is human to have fears and worries, if they show reasonable concern for their child's well-being, the child may come to them for help and reassurance. A friendly talk can substantially reduce a child's fears. Talking to his parents helps make him feel less lonely and therefore less scared.

Toward Self-Reliance

Middle childhood is the time when parents should encourage independence and self-reliance. One cannot give too much love to an infant, but six-to-eleven-year-old children do not need or like too much overtly expressed affection. Of course, they need parental love and approval, and parental rejection can be harmful to their mental health. However, overprotection stifles them and slows down their progress toward adult self-reliance. Many cases of agoraphobia and school phobia (see Sections 1 and 52) are caused by inappropriate parental attitudes.

When a child complains about school, peers, teachers, or any other threatening situation, parents should keep direct intervention to a minimum of absolutely necessary cases. It is imperative to encourage the child to handle his problems on his own. He should be urged to communicate his failures and victories and always made to feel that his parents will not let him down.

Chapter VII.
Adolescence

Adolescents usually outgrow most of their childhood fears. Most adolescents' fears are related to the fact that while they are no longer children and resent being treated as such, neither are they adults. Quite often they act in a childlike manner and they can't help being aware that they still depend on their parents.

The period of transition from infancy to adulthood is prolonged in modern societies. In the past (and today among primitive tribes) puberty rites were designed as a test of adulthood, and the young who passed them were immediately admitted to the community of adults. As adults, they were expected to earn their own living, marry, and support a family. Socio-cultural maturity and physical maturity were expected to coincide. In the ancient Jewish tradition the Bar Mitzvah ceremony signaled the beginning of responsibility. Until the age of thirteen the boy's sins were blamed on his father, but from this age on the boy was held responsible for his actions.

The transition from childhood to adulthood is not an easy task in any society but the complexity of modern societies creates additional difficulties for the youth. The age of physical maturation has not changed much over the millennia, but the concept of psychosocial maturity has undergone substantial alteration.

Physical and sexual maturity are attained today at the age of fifteen to eighteen for boys and thirteen to sixteen for girls, but modern adolescents are neither able to support themselves nor are capable of assuming responsibility for family relationships. A technological society has no use for juvenile shepherds and hunters—the modern economic system is based on skilled labor and highly qualified managerial and professional cadres. A high-school dropout can hardly earn a living in our society, and there are fewer and fewer job opportunities for unskilled labor. Prolonged schooling is therefore necessary for economic reasons, and adequate psychocultural maturity is a prerequisite for adult participation in modern societies. Such socio-economic-cultural maturity requires a high level of psychological development, which can hardly be attained in the teens.

This discrepancy between bio-psychological and socio-cultural maturity is aggravated by several factors. One is inherent in the glandular and other biochemical changes adolescents undergo, which are accompanied by added physical and mental energy, aggressiveness, and frequent overestimation of their own potentialities. The adolescent and postadolescent years are a period of frequent conflicts, for young people tend to believe that they are adult and therefore should be granted the status of adults.

PSYCHOLOGY OF CHILDREN'S FEARS

This process of self-assertion leads to a normal breaking away from parental authority. In early adolescence children take the first step in this rebellion; in their late teens and postadolescence they take the second step. Usually the first step is wholly negative. Adolescents seem to be trying to do whatever is contrary to parental wishes. They intentionally break parental rules and indulge in juvenile pranks intended to show their independence, all the while depending on their parents economically and psychologically.

Identity Problems

Many adolescents experience intense anxiety over their sense of self and identity. Only yesterday they were children, but now they are physically grown, sexually mature, and on the threshold of adult life. They ask themselves, "Who am I—a child or a grown-up man or woman?" They are afraid to admit that they fear to become adults, and resent anyone who tells them that truth. Sometimes they wish to continue as children, and this is a most embarrassing admission. Small wonder that many adolescents display an astounding lack of fear. This bravado is a cover for nagging doubts about their ability to face the responsibilities of adulthood.

Fears of self-reproach, of inadequacy, of being a failure, of not being able to cope with sexual and economic problems are common in adolescents. Their dependence on parental approval declines, but since they have not yet developed self-reliance, they tend to depend on their peers. Many adolescents fear disapproval and rejection by their peer group far more than parental disapproval.

Preadolescents and adolescents form close-knit cliques that offer them the security they do not possess on their own. Even though juvenile groups and gangs can be far more demanding than parents, it is painfully difficult for an adolescent to admit that he needs the "old generation" for protection from their despotism.

Belonging to a clique, group, or gang gives teenagers a most enjoyable feeling of power, albeit a false one. Protected by membership in the group, they do things they wouldn't do as individuals. Their antisocial behavior is a product of disappearance of the normal fear of potentially dangerous consequences.

Psychosexual Identity

Adolescents are big and tall and do not fear darkness, loud noises, bogeymen, and separation, but typically they are unsure of their ability to stand on their own and meet the challenges of life. Thus they suffer more from anxiety than from fear. Their main anxieties concern their present peer relationships and future adult roles.

Adolescent anxieties are most often related to psychosexual identification. The questions "Who am I" and "Where am I going" hinge on the desire to be "a real man" or "a real woman." Sexuality means much more than physiological gratification. It encompasses self-image as an adult, self-esteem, and success with the opposite sex.

Sexual relations start in interaction with another person who is a potential sexual partner. Dating requires a certain degree of courage, both for boys and girls. Some adolescents disguise their anxiety with bravado, but many avoid even initial contact with the opposite sex out of fear of sounding stupid or looking ugly and being rejected.

The intense adolescent sexual urge often creates fear and anxiety about the size and appearance of primary and secondary sexual characteristics and about the ability to perform. Many adolescent boys believe that their penis is

PSYCHOLOGY OF CHILDREN'S FEARS

too small. A nineteen-year-old patient explained to me that he couldn't date girls because his penis was atrophied, a condition he believed he had brought on by masturbation. Obviously, his conviction was not true and, after a period of psychoanalytic psychotherapy, he began to date and to sleep with girls. His story was a cover-up for his fear of women and sexual impotence, related to his unresolved Oedipus complex.

Some adolescent boys fear they cannot satisfy a woman. Some dread early ejaculation, others homosexual inclinations. Adolescent girls may worry about the size of their vaginal tracts and fear that their insides are too small to hold a penis or a baby.

Sexual fears are rarely if ever related to physiology. They almost certainly reflect a lack of self-confidence. The absence of faith in oneself affects most aspects of human behavior, and especially the sensitive area of psychosexual identity and sexual relations.

Reaction Formation

Shy, withdrawn preadolescents and adolescents are prone to develop school phobia (see Section 52) or agoraphobia (see Section 1). The appearance of a phobia can be precipitated by a traumatic event, but usually such aversions grow slowly. A young boy who is not popular with girls because he is overly sensitive or shy, and who desperately craves feminine company, may suddenly develop a feeling diametrically opposed to what he originally felt. Actually he is tremendously attracted to girls, but because he believes that he has no chance with any of them, he begins to hate all of them. This psychological mechanism, called reaction formation, serves as a cover-up for his true feelings and artificially protects his self-esteem. "Who needs these stupid girls," he brags. He wishes to punish all of them in revenge against the one or two who rejected his clumsy advances. He fears that if once he puts his hands on any girl, he will lose all self-control. Result: agoraphobia. His fear of open spaces will prevent him from attacking girls because it compels him to seek the company of another person whose presence will inhibit his impulses.

Many adolescents who doubt their sexual identity try to overcome their anxiety by hectic sexual behavior. Thus, a shy and anxious girl may act in a sexually aggressive and excessively promiscuous manner, and a boy who doubts his masculinity may brag about the number of girls he has "made."

Escape into Addiction

Fear of being a helpless weakling drives some adolescents into totally irrational behavior. Excessive craving for alcohol or drugs is usually a double-edged sword. On the one hand, it helps an adolescent mask his fears and anxieties. Getting "high" or "stoned" makes him feel uninhibited, fearless, and powerful. Since this imaginary power does not last too long, there is a continuous need to renew and increase the dosage.

In reality, alcohol and drugs make people less powerful. The feeling of power they induce is an illusion, and after the "high," the adolescent is even more aware of his deep weakness. Unable to cope with this self-knowledge, he becomes more and more dependent on the drug or drink that allows him to forget his weakness—he escapes into addiction.

Alcohol and drug abuse are serious problems and in practically all cases they require professional help. However, parental concern and understanding can have a most

PSYCHOLOGY OF CHILDREN'S FEARS

beneficial effect. In some instances the parents could have prevented their occurrence, and in all cases of professional intervention parental cooperation is of utmost importance for successful therapy.

Alcohol and drug abuse affects children of every social class and economic level. It is a widespread phenomenon in our high schools and colleges, and even in the higher grades of some elementary schools. Rarely does it start at home, but if the parents themselves are alcoholics or drug addicts, the chances are that their children will follow in their footsteps. Parental preaching and moralizing have little effect, for, as usual, actions speak louder than words.

I had in treatment several youngsters afflicted to various degrees with alcoholism and drug addiction. One of them attended a private school where he was the chief drug pusher. Another boy attended a rigorous parochial school, and both his parents were devoted churchgoers. A severely addicted girl was the daughter of a school principal. Still another was the daughter of a business executive and a feminist leader. In short, addicted adolescents come from all sorts of homes and can pick up their habit at a progressive or a traditional school.

Our society has its share of criminal drug pushers who make a living poisoning our youth, but the fact that so many youngsters are an easy prey makes one realize that there is widespread susceptibility to pathological behavior.

All forms of addiction are clearly pathological, for they violate the fundamental law of human life, which is self-preservation. The fear of harming one's health and the avoidance of self-destruction are common to all mentally healthy people, young and old alike.

All the youngsters I have treated for various addictions knew they were harming themselves, but either they

CHILDREN'S FEARS

were unable to resist temptation or they were too far gone to use good judgment. Some of them made up excuses for their behavior; others maintained their bodies could take any poison.

In dealing with this grave problem one should avoid simplistic generalizations. Every case is different—every parent and every adolescent are particular persons. One must take into consideration a host of cultural and psychological factors and look for the particular factors that motivated the adolescent to seek this morbid escape from life.

There is, however, one common denominator: *All addicts seek escape from torturous feelings of inferiority, inadequacy, weakness, hopelessness, and depression. Practically all of them perceive themselves as unable to cope with their problems, be they sexual, academic, or any other kind. They lack the courage to face life head on; they doubt their own resources and don't believe that anyone is willing to and/or capable of helping them. In the vast majority of cases addiction is an act of despair.*

The following descriptions will attest to the diversity of background and similarity of psychological motivation in addicts.

My patient, an energetic businesswoman married to a bright but rather ineffectual and subservient man, brought to my office her fifteen-year-old son. The boy attended a private school but nevertheless managed to associate with what his mother called "the scum of the earth" in his neighborhood. He was drinking heavily and often treated his friends to booze. One evening when the parents came home from the theater, they found their son giving a party for a bunch of boys and girls, some of whom were quite drunk.

When the boy was caught shoplifting and stealing, his

father bawled him out and then hired lawyers to prove his son's innocence. The boy told me that in the private school he attended he was "the last man on the totem pole and no one respected him." But in the neighborhood he was a "big shot" and his drinking friends were his "bodyguards."

The boy was physically small and rather timid. He could never depend on his father, whom he described as his mother's "servant." The mother, said the boy, "wiped the floor with the old man," who was constantly interrupted and overruled by his wife. Once when the boy told his father that he had been beaten up in school, the father told him to ask his mother's help and advice.

Drinking gave the boy the feeling of power he craved. It made him feel strong and brave, and under the influence of alcohol he began to do brazen things. He talked down to the "poor slobs" in the neighborhood and bossed them around. When intoxicated, he could even stand up to his mother and call her dirty names. Once his mother threatened that she would ask his father to punish him and the boy laughed in her face. Liquor gave him "a great feeling" and without it, he said, he would feel lonely and helpless.

In adolescence drug addiction is more frequent than alcoholism, and I would like to describe the case of a fourteen-year-old girl brought by her parents for consultation because she was "cutting classes and playing hookie." Her father gave me a lengthy lecture on discipline and moral ideals. His wife nodded with what looked like forced approval. She did not say a word except "Good morning, Doctor" and "So long, Doctor." The father spoke incessantly, spouting clichés.

It took a while before I won the girl's confidence so she would speak freely to me. Her home life was a nightmare. Her father was generally a rather meek man, but occasionally he lost his temper and asserted himself in a violent manner. Every so often he murderously beat his wife, accusing her of infidelity, of spending too much money, of mismanaging the household, and so on. Most of the time he obeyed his wife's orders, but whenever they disagreed, their discussions ended in a verbal and physical fight and the mother was usually badly bruised.

The mother took revenge on the children. My patient and her older sister, who was hospitalized after overdosing, were physically punished for the slightest transgressions. My fourteen-year-old patient felt like a caged animal, trapped inside a home where she was subjected to frequent maternal and occasional paternal violence. She felt that no one cared for her, and her use of a variety of drugs (whatever she could get) was an escape into a world of imaginary security, peace, and happiness.

Her girlfriend's parents worked. My patient and a few boys and girls frequently gathered in the basement in the mornings, shared drugs, and practiced indiscriminate sexual relations.

Drug addiction is usually a symptom of deeper emotional problems, the smoke that indicates the fire of deep-rooted anxiety.

One of the saddest of my cases was a nineteen-year-old boy who was arrested as a "drug pusher." His parents got him off and brought him to my office. Both of them were in tears because they could not believe this had happened to their child.

The mother and father were prominent civic leaders in their suburban community. Both served on the board of the local church and both were conscientious, responsible, and intelligent people.

Unfortunately, they did not pay adequate attention to

PSYCHOLOGY OF CHILDREN'S FEARS

their son. They believed that *their* ideas and ideals would protect him from doing wrong and getting into trouble. When he called them from the police station and told them he had been arrested, they couldn't believe it. When they were told that he had been selling drugs, they were profoundly shocked.

They were totally unaware that their son, an amiable, charming, and bright boy, for years had suffered severely from feelings of inferiority and anxiety and was frequently depressed. In childhood he had been skinny, fragile, and frequently bedridden with a variety of respiratory diseases. His peers ridiculed him, refused to admit him to their ball games, and often ganged up on him. His father could not understand his son, or cared not to, and often criticized his "sissy" behavior. His mother was a rigid disciplinarian who lived by the book and refused to see reality. The boy felt lonely, misunderstood, and terribly inadequate. His mother decided that what this shy and insecure boy needed was stern discipline, so she sent him to a tough boarding school far from home and the few friends he had. She exposed him to a rigid discipline he was unable to take.

At that school he became friendly with other boys who were failing subjects. He himself failed both academic subjects and physical education. He feared his teachers and peers and found escape in uppers and downers and became seriously addicted.

I have had in treatment several other youngsters addicted to drugs and a few who were alcoholics. They were sixteen to twenty years old, the majority of them college students, and suffering from insecurity, loneliness, and fear of facing life.

Children and adolescents do not have enough power to face alone the hardships of their developmental years.

CHILDREN'S FEARS

They need parental support and encouragement. Understanding, friendly, considerate parents, who at the same time can be firm and set limits, create an atmosphere conducive to wholesome growth. Should their son or daughter experiment with drugs, they can stop it immediately by a stern warning and by showing concern for the youngster's physical and mental health. Parents who evoke love and fear of disapproval do not need to use force; their children obey them without threats or punishments (see Chapter VIII, Do's and Don'ts for Parents).

Parents must find out what made their son or daughter seek escape in drugs. What bothers them, what are they afraid of, what kind of fear are they trying to escape from. As long as the parents are perceived by their children as friendly but not wishy-washy, as long as they are loved, respected, and trusted, they have a good chance of preventing drug abuse. One of my patients successfully handled a danger-fraught situation. Her fifteen-year-old daughter was acting strangely and the mother sensed that she was experimenting with drugs. She explained the dangers to her daughter. She was quite firm, but at the same time tried to understand why her timid daughter needed to compensate for her anxiety by joining a drug-using crowd, and she successfully guided the girl.

In practically all cases drug abuse requires professional help, but parental firmness and unswerving trust can prevent a great many troubles. Parents must not increase their children's fears and worries by distrust, harshness, and punishment. Neither should they give their children the feeling that they don't care what they do. Permissiveness is most often perceived as abandonment, and confirms the adolescent's feeling that no one cares about him, that he is alone with his fears and worries, and that there is no point in confiding in his parents.

PSYCHOLOGY OF CHILDREN'S FEARS

Dealing with Adolescent Fears

It is not easy for parents to handle adolescent fears mainly because many adolescents perceive their parents as being friendly but weak (see Chapter I). This lack of respect for parents reduces the chances of parental help.

Alleviating adolescent fears depends on parental ability to cope with adolescents. Parents must not renounce their power and acceptance position until their children reach maturity. Adolescents seek the advice of parents they perceive as strong and friendly, parents they can respect and depend on.

Though parents must offer help when necessary, their main task is to encourage independence and self-reliance. They must treat adolescent boys and girls not as children but as grownups, encourage their work, and solicit and respect their judgment.

Chapter VIII.
Do's and Don'ts for Parents

Parents are not omnipotent, but their attitudes and actions can favorably or adversely affect their children's fears. As explained in Chapters I and II, the child initially borrows his security from parental love and protection. As he grows older, stronger, and more self-reliant, his sense of security becomes more related to his own power.

The present chapter discusses the role of parents. It starts with a description of what parents must not do and ends with advice on what they can and should do.

Scaring the Child

Scaring a scared child is tantamount to pouring oil on fire. Parents can set limits to a child's behavior without aggravating his fears and making him more insecure.

If a child must be warned against transgressing parental rules and informed of the consequences of his

PSYCHOLOGY OF CHILDREN'S FEARS

deeds, the warning should be short, precise, and concrete. A warning represents a threat, and a threat can be useful if it helps prevent inappropriate and antisocial behavior. But threats must be implemented or they are useless and even harmful. A threat that is not carried out teaches the child to disrespect his parents and disturbs his normal growth. The nature of the threat is also important. Such threats as "You will not be allowed to watch TV until you finish your homework" have a limited use, but threatening the child with being abandoned can create an unhealthy panic state.

A child can adjust to fair and strict parents. If he loves and respects them, there will be no need for punishment. Vague threats and too generalized ones adversely affect the child's feeling of security and unnecessarily elicit additional fears. Children take parental communication literally, and they are in no position to know that their neck will still be in one piece after a mother threatens, "I will break your neck." They may not know the meaning of the word "pulp," but it sounds terrible indeed when an angry father shouts, "I will beat you to a pulp!"

Some parents aggravate the child's fear. One five-year-old who feared darkness was told that if he refused to finish his heaping bowl of oatmeal, he would be locked in a dark room together "with the monsters who live there and hide under the furniture."

Forcing an agoraphobic child to go outdoors or pushing a child who fears dogs to face a big growling dog is to precipitate an attack of anxiety or worse.

In *Child Psychology*, p. 332, Dr. A. T. Jersild reported a story told to him by a six-year-old boy:

> His mother had told him that because he had been bad (he had quarreled with his sister) a time would come when he could not be able to move the hand that struck his sister. The mother then described what happened to

a neighbor's child. The child died, the mother said, and he was put in a coffin. But his hand remained outside the coffin, and no one could put it inside. The lid of the coffin could not be closed until a priest had struck the hand and then it slipped into the coffin. Meanwhile, his mother said, everyone talked about this child, and laughed and laughed, *and this may also happen to you.*

Expressing Fears

Many parents discourage children from expressing their fears. They seem to believe that suppressed emotions cease to exist, and disapprove or even ridicule a child who tells them he or she is scared. Every so often a parent will react angrily to a frightened child and says something like: "Other boys don't fear bugs. It's only you, sissy!" Or "Girls your age have long outgrown their stupid fears!" Or "When I was your age I did not fear being left alone!"

Needless to say, such an attitude does not help the child and might aggravate his fears. The child does not lose his original fear, and an additional burden has been added—he now also fears parental rejection.

Undue Permissiveness

Overly permissive parents don't teach their children to be aware of the realistic consequences of their behavior. Because they refuse to set limits they do not give their children the opportunity to develop adequate self-control. Children have an inadequate perception of reality; sometimes they don't fear the things they should fear and do fear nondangerous things. Parental guidance is an absolute prerequisite for normal child development.

Moreover, parents who are too lenient undermine the child's feeling of security. Normally, the child perceives his parents as being strong and friendly—that is, possessing

PSYCHOLOGY OF CHILDREN'S FEARS

the power necessary to protect him and determined to use it in his defense. The child looks up to his parents, trusts them, and tries to follow them, but undecided, overly permissive parents do not inspire confidence. The child feels that their constant giving in proves how weak they are.

Inconsistency

A child has a reasonably good chance to adjust to parents who are conservative or progressive, religious or atheistic, very neat or rather sloppy, but finds it difficult to adjust to changing and unpredictable demands. Inconsistent parents force a child to live in constant fear of disapproval and punishment, and blame himself for not being able to comply with their self-contradictory demands.

Overdemanding Attitudes

Sometimes well-wishing parents expect too much from their child and unwillingly and unwittingly create anxiety. Every child wants to please his parents and live up to their expectations, but parents who demand too much too soon force their child to overextend himself and live in constant fear of "failing" his parents.

Setting too high or unattainable goals is the royal road to anxiety and frustration. An "overdemanded" child worries continually. He also tends to underestimate his achievements, for no matter how well he does at something today, he fears he may not do as well tomorrow and hurt his parents' feelings.

Involving the Child

There is no ideal, universally valid child-rearing method. A child can be well brought up by brilliant or by average parents, by active and dynamic or by slow and passive ones, as long as they care for the child and don't involve him in their problems.

No parent feeds an infant solid food before the child is ready for it, or gives him a piece of apple before he can bite, chew, and digest. The same rule applies to emotional food. No child should be exposed to emotions he cannot comprehend or cope with.

No human life is free of hardships, challenges, threats, and frustrations, so no parent can always be a smiling, cheerful angel. Most children are quite sturdy and can adjust to their parents' moods, but they should not be compelled to become their parents' partners, confessors, or protectors.

Parents have the right and obligation to impose their rules on their children, but they have no right or reason to impose their worries, fears, and anxieties on them. Children cannot solve parental problems—they cannot find a job for an unemployed father, they cannot stop the Internal Revenue Service from collecting income tax, they cannot fix a broken washing machine, they cannot prevent a grandmother from getting sick, and they cannot make their parents love each other. They must be allowed to live their own life, facing *their* age-level problems, and to grow and develop according to *their* biological rhythm.

Don't Rush

Not every child develops at the same speed, and early growth is not necessarily a sign of superiority, nor slow growth an indication of mental retardation. Many toddlers, for instance, derive a great deal of pleasure from prolonged finger sucking. Usually this desire gradually diminishes and then disappears. Some parents seem to believe they can regulate their child's developmental rhythm and worry if it does not conform to the statistical averages.

I once had in treatment a fifty-year-old successful businessman who sucked his thumb whenever he felt upset. His thumb-sucking obsession went back to his very early years when his mother decided that he was falling behind the statistical developmental schedules and that he might become mentally defective. To prevent finger sucking, she tied his hands and he learned not to suck in her presence. However, whenever he was tired, sleepy, or upset, he reverted to finger sucking, which created profound anxiety.

Disapproval

It is not wrong to be cross with a misbehaving child. Parents who express their disapproval or anger at a child's behavior help the child to develop *normal fears*. They teach him the cause-and-effect relationship between human actions and their outcome. It is necessary at times to disapprove of a child's particular behavior, but parents should *never disapprove of the child.* They must set limits, but at the same time they must show their love and affection. They must be strong and friendly.

Resenting the Child

All parents occasionally resent their children because children reduce one's freedom. Moreover, their behavior can be irritating and, not too infrequently, drive even the most patient parent up the wall.

Admitting to oneself that one is angry usually alleviates the anger. Of course, mature parents do not indiscriminately *act out* their anger. Their love for and understanding of their child enables them to react rationally even in difficult situations.

CHILDREN'S FEARS

There is a great difference between control of actions and control of emotions. Control of actions is a sign of maturity, but control or denial of emotions leads to inner tension. Parents who deny that they are, occasionally, quite annoyed at their child are likely to develop inner conflicts. Some of them feel guilty for resenting the child's misbehavior and in order to appease their guilt become overprotective.

Why Some Parents Overprotect Their Child

Children's mental health is closely connected to their feeling of security—that is, of being loved and protected. Hatred and rejection are certainly worse than overprotection, but neither extreme does the child any good.

For one thing, overprotection does not prove parental love. Overprotecting parents may pronounce great love and may even believe that their anxious overprotective actions are generated by love for their child, but this is rarely if ever true.

The message an overprotected child gets is very simple: "Your mother and/or father don't trust you. They don't believe you can accomplish anything on your own. They think you are helpless, clumsy, and not too bright."

Suppose a little child wants to climb on a chair. A wise parent watches him and encourages his efforts. Success builds self-confidence, and the child is encouraged to cope with hardships. The parent stands by to be of help only if absolutely necessary. Should the child fail, the parent encourages further efforts. The child feels that the father or mother has faith in him and will help if needed.

To love a child means helping him to grow into a self-confident, mature adult. Overprotecting parents prevent such a growth. They infantilize the child.

PSYCHOLOGY OF CHILDREN'S FEARS

Parental overprotection puts the child down and undermines his self-confidence and therefore increases his fear. The overprotected child may develop feelings of inferiority and inadequacy and become overattached and overdependent on his parents.

The Role of Parents

Many children experience two conflicting tendencies. On the one hand, they wish to grow and do what grownups do, but on the other hand, they wish to remain helpless children who can count on help from without. Anxious children wish to remain children because they don't trust themselves and fear adult responsibility.

Ultimately a child must be helped to outgrow childhood and become a mature person. Mature people are capable of realistically assessing potential dangers and their own resources, and of acting accordingly. They do not hide from imaginary dangers nor are they are given to hysterical panic. They are reasonably brave; they accept challenge and take calculated risks. They do not indulge in wishful thinking that someone will save them nor do they regress into feeling sorry for themselves.

Mature adults are not fearless fools either. They neither underestimate hardships nor overestimate their own power. They experience normal, realistic fears and act upon them in an adjustive, self-preserving manner. Mature adults can stand alone but relate to other people to increase their own security and power and contribute the same to their allies.

Parents can help their child to overcome his fears and phobias, provided they are aware of his fears and present themselves as both strong and friendly. Being strong implies dependability, decisiveness, and self-confidence, but strength can be used to help or to hurt and parents must convey a friendly, caring attitude in words and deeds.

It is very important to find out what the *child can do for himself,* how he can develop the ability to cope with stress and threats and master difficult situations. The aim of parental care and education is to make that care and education superfluous, to help the child cease to be a child and become a well-adjusted adult.

Setting an Example

Fear and courage are psychologically contagious. Both emotions can be communicated both verbally or nonverbally. Primitive warriors beat drums and sing or play heroic tunes to encourage their comrades. Pep talks and patriotic martial songs greatly contribute to combat bravery.

At the same time frightening noises and panic-inducing rumors undermine courage. Fear is closely related to a low estimate of one's own powers and the powers of one's allies (see Chapter I). Panic spreads as fast as a forest fire, and the fear of one small unit in combat may cause mass panic and bring a serious defeat to a large army.

A child who fears darkness will be greatly encouraged by the parent who takes his hand and gently shows him around a dark room. A child who fears water must not be pushed into large ocean waves, but may be guided into a swimming pool. Seeing his parents wading in not-too-deep waters may considerably reduce his fears.

Expression of Fear

As a rule, it is better for the child to express his fears and anxieties openly than to hide them. Children who are embarrassed, shamed, and ridiculed into denying their fears are deprived of the best method of coping with them.

PSYCHOLOGY OF CHILDREN'S FEARS

An imaginary fear can best be handled by a tactful *reality test*. A child who fears darkness in his own bedroom should be helped to check the room in full light. A child who fears mirrors, vacuum cleaners, and other objects should be shown by a friendly adult that all these things are harmless.

Realistic fears should be coped with in a rational way. If a child fears crossing the street, he should be helped and guided in paying full attention to traffic lights and taught to cross on the green light only.

It is much better if a child remembers what frightened him and is reassured and encouraged to cope with it. "Forgetting" does not lead to overcoming a fear, for in most cases the fear remains in the subconscious and returns in a more frightening form in dreams or displaced fears called phobias.

Encouragement

Some children's fears gradually disappear by themselves. A study of phobic preschool children discovered that after five years all of them had substantially improved, and in some the phobia had completely disappeared.

Since fear is related to one's estimate of one's own power in comparison to the power of the threatening person, animal, or situation, the less one thinks of one's own power, the more one is prone to fear. As the child grows bigger and stronger, he has less reason to fear. Thus, for instance, the fear of darkness diminishes with age.

However, people's actions are determined not by the objective situation but by the way they *perceive* it. A big, strong child might fear little puppies if he believes in the puppy's power and his own helplessness. To have power is important, but unless one is aware of one's own power, he may not be able to use it. In other words, parents and teachers must *encourage the child* and make him aware of his ability to cope with certain dangers. The cowardly lion in *The Wizard of Oz* was certainly powerful, but badly underestimated his own power and overestimated the power of potential threats.

Some psychologists maintain that fear can spur motivation, at least in school situations. A child who fears bad marks or other punishment will try harder, they reason. Undoubtedly, this incentive works with *some* children but certainly not with all. Shy and timid children who are threatened with punishment and anticipate defeat may become more discouraged and lose whatever faith they had in themselves. This may make them give up trying altogether.

Encouragement is a far better method of coping with a child's fears than discouragement, and rewards are a stronger motivation than punishment.

Overdoing

Though children need encouragement, an exaggerated dose of it may cause more harm than good. To insist forcefully that a frightened little boy or girl pet a threatening German shepherd is not advisable. Only an immature father or mother wishes to boast to friends about such a heroic child. And if the dog barks, or even worse, snaps, the little hero may panic and burst into tears and develop a severe dog phobia.

The right attitude is based on a realistic appraisal of what the child is psychologically ready to do.

Children must be guided to cope with dangerous situations in an *active* rather than *passive* manner. Passivity deepens one's feeling of weakness and helplessness, and thus increases one's fears. Active, aggressive behavior in-

PSYCHOLOGY OF CHILDREN'S FEARS

creases one's faith in one's own powers, and children should be taught to *master dangers rather than retreat from them.*

Major Dangers

There is nothing wrong in admitting realistic fears. Parents who hide their fears in wartime or other disasters are likely to either communicate their fear nonverbally or make their children feel lonely. Nonverbally communicated fear increases the child's own fear, for God only knows how bad things are if parents are scared to admit that they too are afraid. Successfully masked fear, on the other hand, may give the child the uncomfortable feeling that he is the only coward and is open to ridicule.

Realistic admission of fear by the parents leaves room for coping with dangers in a rational way and creates in a child the feeling of belonging. In times of war, floods, earthquakes, and so on, the children should be made aware of parental fears and allowed to take part in whatever has to be done.

Building the Child's Self-Reliance

The awareness of his own gradually growing power plays an important role in the way the child learns to overcome his fears. Just yesterday he was three feet tall, but today, Mommy, see how big I am! Children continually measure and compare. They ask, Who is stronger, the lion or the tiger? The elephant or the rhinoceros? Or, who is smarter, prettier, wealthier, and so on.

Children take pride in their growing strength and motor agility. The more faith they have in their own power, the easier it is for them to overcome their fears.

CHILDREN'S FEARS

In summary:

Don't *1.* Don't ignore the child's fears; don't dismiss them.

2. Don't overprotect the child; avoid making him feel helpless and overdependent on you; don't pity him.

3. Don't reject the child. Don't threaten him with abandonment; don't make him feel lonely.

4. Don't ridicule the fearful child. Don't punish him for being afraid.

5. Don't force the child into a situation he fears.

6. Don't involve your child in your own fears.

Do *1.* Build the child's faith in himself and his abilities.

2. Praise his achievements, no matter how small they are (but without exaggeration).

3. Make him feel that you will always love him and protect him whenever necessary.

4. Listen patiently to the child and show understanding for his fears; whenever possible, try to explain that there is nothing to be afraid of.

5. Set an example by rationally coping with dangers yourself.

6. Give the child the opportunity to overcome his fears actively.

Part Two
Children's Fears
in Alphabetical
Order

CHILDREN'S FEARS IN ALPHABETICAL ORDER

CHILDREN'S FEARS IN ALPHABETICAL ORDER

CHILDREN'S FEARS IN ALPHABETICAL ORDER

SECTION 1. *Agoraphobia*

Agoraphobia, an intense fear of open spaces, is a combination of two distinct fears, namely the fear of being alone and the fear of leaving the familiar and presumably safe home environment. The fear of leaving home seems to be the major factor in agoraphobia; however, many agoraphobic children are less afraid to go outdoors when accompanied by a friendly person.

Agoraphobia is not a frequent phenomenon in children. Usually it starts either at school age or adolescence. Agoraphobia is often precipitated by severe illness of the child himself or by an illness or bereavement in the family, but its true causes lie in the child's unconscious feelings and wishes.

Often agoraphobia is a displacement of hostile feelings toward parents or a fear of one's own hostile impulses. Psychologists, psychiatrists, and psychoanalysts have frequently written about a child who hates his parents, most often his mother, and stays home to protect her against his own hostile impulses.

Sometimes shy and timid adolescent boys develop a hatred of girls. They rationalize that girls reject them, while actually they defeat themselves by clumsy advances or by a paralyzing fear of approaching girls. Obsessed by unconscious sexual and/or aggressive impulses, they fear they may not be able to control themselves and that they will assault the woman they fear, hate, and desire all at the same time.

Children tend to take parental words literally, and a parent's transient hardship may be perceived by a child as impending doom. When a mother says to her frugal husband, "I'd rather kill myself than go to the Joneses in the same dress they saw me in the last time," a child may worry about his mother's suicide and wish to stay home to prevent this catastrophe.

Agoraphobia can also be induced by parents who unwittingly (and most often nonverbally) convey to the child the notion that *they* feel lonely and need the child's physical presence to allay their fears and anxieties. Sometimes a woman who has lost her husband clings to her school-age or adolescent son or daughter. The child then refuses to go out because he worries about his poor, lonely mother and/or feels guilty when he leaves her home alone. The child may develop a persistent fear of going out and, unaware of his true feelings, believe that he is simply afraid to be in open spaces. Most often his fear is a displaced expression of role reversal: he worries about his parent, instead of the parent worrying about him. I once had in treatment an adolescent girl who developed severe agoraphobia after the death of her mother. The father was a lonely, depressed man, and the girl was afraid to leave him alone.

Agoraphobic children often do not speak of their fear of leaving home but rather of their desire to stay with mother. As with school phobia, the agoraphobic child worries about his mother, and sometimes father. Illness or a death in the family aggravates his worries, and his agoraphobia is a displaced fear substituting for the fear that something terrible will happen at home in his absence.

The symptoms associated with agoraphobia closely resemble those related to school phobia (see Section 52). Agoraphobic children are usually timid, withdrawn, quite depressèd, and suffer a variety of psychosomatic symptoms such as headaches, nausea, loss of appetite, and sleep disturbances.

In many instances agoraphobia requires professional help, but a radical change in parental attitude often produces a miraculous cure. A youngster who is afraid to leave his mother alone may lose his fear of open spaces when his mother begins to act in a self-assured way.

SECTION 2. *Anxiety*

It is not easy to distinguish fear from anxiety, but unrealistic fears often represent inner conflict rather than fear of an external threat. Fear of "bad people" who may break into a well-guarded and well-protected house and "hurt daddy" may be realistic if father is a member of the Mafia and has received phone threats. But if there is no realistic reason to expect unusual acts of violence and vengeance, the child's fears may be an expression of his *own* hostile feelings toward his father and the fear that his wishes may come true. His anxiety is a sign of inner conflict; it is a fear of his own thoughts and wishes.

If a child who has been doing well in school and has excellent marks is suddenly afraid of failing; he is actually expressing a fear of success and a wish to fail. He may be torn between his wish to succeed and fear that his success will elicit more demands from his parents. One of my patients, a high-school boy, cautiously avoided high marks in school because every good mark he received made his parents expect the highest marks in all subjects.

Anxiety states are indicative of overall feelings of helplessness and worthlessness. Fear is a temporary reaction to danger. Anxiety is a prolonged state of tension and apprehension. Anxious children, expecting impending doom, become irritable, afraid to take the initiative, gloomy, and unproductive. Anxiety often causes loss of appetite, disturbed sleep, nightmares, and other psychosomatic symptoms.

Some irrational fears are actually anxiety states, indicative of an inner conflict. When a child is afraid to fall asleep, it may be because he fears bad dreams. The bad dreams reflect his inner conflicts. A six-year-old girl who was afraid to go to sleep intensely hated her two-week-old baby brother. For six years she had enjoyed all her parents' attention and after the birth of the baby she felt neglected and rejected. She was told by her parents that she was supposed to love her brother, but she did not feel much sisterly love and felt guilty. Apparently, she wasn't a "nice little girl," though she tried to display affection for the baby. At night she was plagued by nightmares.

A child who feels unloved by his parents may blame himself for the rejection. Disparaging remarks, destructive criticism, and frequent and harsh punishment contribute to the child's feeling of anxiety and worthlessness. Exaggerated parental demands may produce anxiety states in a child who feels he can never live up to the standards set by his parents. The best way to prevent your child from becoming anxious is to give him the feeling that you love him and will always protect him. You may disapprove of some of his behavior, but you never disapprove of him. A child who feels accepted and secure is not an anxious child.

SECTION 3. *Fear of Abandonment*

As explained in the first two chapters, human beings derive their feeling of security from two sources: their own power and the loyalty and power of their allies. The child's own power is negligible; the younger he is, the less power he has. His feeling of security depends on the power of his parents and their willingness to use it to protect him. Abandonment is therefore the worst thing that can happen to a child, for his supply of food and his very survival depend on parental care.

It is not enough for a child to get food now. His security depends on his confidence that the food and protection will be forthcoming in the future. The newborn child is endowed with the ability to perceive nonverbal signals and feel whether or not he is loved by the feeding mother or maternal substitute. This ability, called *empathy,* imbues the infant with feelings of security and euphoria, or fear and anxiety. Infants need to be loved, and they are blissfully happy when the feeding mother hugs, kisses, and speaks affectionately to them. When the feeding mother resents the child and thinks how great her life could be without the baby, the child empathizes her feelings and becomes anxiety ridden. He clings to his mother because he does not trust her and fears she will abandon him.

If a mother works outside the home, this does not necessarily harm the child's mental health. A mother may go to work every day and leave the child with a trusted person, provided the child is sure the mother will come back at a certain time. Infants do not need clocks; they follow their own biological time clock. Parental dependability reduces the displeasure of temporary separation, and as long as the child can trust his mother's love, he can accept her absence and relate well to the grandmother, nurse, or babysitter who substitutes for her.

It cannot be stressed often enough that though parents may occasionally disapprove of their child's behavior. they should *never disapprove of the child himself* or threaten him with abandonment. They may say, even harshly, "I don't like your messing up the living room," or (to an older child) "You are not allowed to eat with your fingers; here are the fork and the knife," but they must convey with words and deeds that they are both strong *and* friendly. The child who receives this message will love and trust his parents and grow into a secure and self-assured adult.

A child threatened with abandonment—"I will give you up for adoption," "I will go away and leave you alone," or, worst of all, "I will kill myself"—is likely to develop severe anxiety. He may fear falling asleep for fear mother may do something terrible if he does not keep an eye on her. He may fear going to school (school phobia) or going outdoors (agoraphobia) to play with other children. He may also develop quite serious emotional problems.

SECTION 4. *Fear of Aggression*

Survival is the fundamental goal of all life, and the fear of aggression is universal, common to human beings and animals. All people fear aggression. Adult men and women fear muggers, kidnappers, and murderers, and in times of war and riots they are even more frightened. Fear of real dangers has survival value and need not be suppressed. Whenever parents admit that they too are afraid in the face of danger, they help their children feel they are not silly kids.

Anna Freud and Dorothy Burlingham worked with children in London during the Blitz. Some parents kept their children, even during the worst air raids, while others sent their children away to the safe countryside. Separation from parents (see Section 37) had a more adverse effect on the children's mental health than German bombs because those parents who refused to evacuate their children gave them a better feeling of security than the kind people in the countryside gave to the evacuated children.

To be alone means to rely on one's own resources, which cannot be expected from a child. Even in adults loneliness (see Section 29) increases fear, and the presence of other people, especially of people believed to be both strong and friendly, makes one feel more safe and secure.

A timid child invites aggression. Bullies rarely attack bullies, but a shy and timid child is an ideal target and scapegoat. Parents and teachers must not criticize or ridicule the timid youngster, for their criticism will deepen his feeling of inferiority and make him even more timid. There are two ways in which adults can contribute to the child's courage. One is by assuring him of their support, and the other is by building his self-confidence. Rational encouragement builds self-confidence, but pushing a child to fight stronger enemies does not.

Outside support need not be limited to parents; it should also include the child's peers. As the child grows, his dependence on his parents decreases and his involvement with his contemporaries increases.

SECTION 5. *Fear of Own Aggressivity*

Children often believe that their good and bad wishes will come true. Many of them are convinced that their bad words or curses can cause harm to their parents. Sometimes children ascribe their own feelings to others, even to inanimate objects. Sometimes they have nightmares full of ferocious beasts and monsters, who represent their own hostile wishes. One of my younger colleagues reported the case of a six-and-a-half-year-old boy who was afraid to go to sleep because he dreamed of "horrible, murderous monsters," who actually represented his intense hostility to his mother and fear of this guilt-provoking feeling.

Another psychoanalyst treated a seven-year-old boy who refused to go to school. His school phobia started suddenly, during a school assembly, when one of the teachers played the piano. A few days earlier one of the neighbors had committed suicide. When the little boy came home from school, he found his parents and neighbors profoundly upset, and he wished he had been home earlier, as if his presence could have prevented the death. Moreover, he had a long-harbored resentment against his mother, who played the piano, and now began to fear that whenever he left home, his unconscious wish for her destruction might come true. The psychoanalyst who treated the boy cleared his phobia when she explained that many children harbor such wishes and fear they may come true, but that there is nothing terribly wrong in these wishes. They are temporary, transient, normal anger reactions, and there is no reason to fear they may come true.

SECTION 6. *Fear of Animals*

Fear of animals usually appears in the third year of life and it is quite frequent up to the eighth or ninth year. It seems to decline somewhat in later childhood and adolescence, but it does not completely disappear, and quite a few adults fear animals, big and small.

Fear of animals may have a realistic origin in threatening encounters with big dogs in the cities, and with horses, bulls, and other animals in farm country. This fear, which makes one cautious in dealing with big animals, may have some survival value, and parents should teach children not to tease or annoy any animal.

Fear of animals, however, is not always related to a realistic appraisal of possible dangers. The fear of small kittens, puppies, rabbits, and other animals who can do no harm may be learned by association. An unrealistic fear of ferocious beasts the child may have seen in a zoo or at the circus or on television is often a symbolic substitute for other fears the child fears more (see Section 51 on phobias).

Fear of small animals can be overcome by combining the sight of them with pleasant experiences, such as holding the child, feeding, or playing. The child will then associate kittens or rabbits with the pleasure derived from playing or being fed.

CHILDREN'S FEARS IN ALPHABETICAL ORDER

SECTION 7. *Fear of Annihilation*

Many two-to-three-year-old children notice how things disappear and fear this could happen to them. They may watch with curiosity, mixed with terror, their own feces being flushed down the toilet bowl. Or they note the disappearance of water in the bathtub and experience a fear of annihilation.

Ridicule will make a fearful infant even more frightened. A little child is unable to draw logical conclusions, but ridicule makes him feel lonely, rejected, and therefore more exposed to true or imaginary dangers. Reassurance is the best way of handling this fear.

SECTION 8. *Fear of the Bath*

Usually, infants like to playfully splash in the bathtub or bathinette, but sometimes they may panic and refuse to take a bath. This fear, however insignificant it seems to a parent, should not be made light of. Quite often the flow of water down the drain throws the infant into a panic. Seeing the water disappear, he may fear the same could happen to him (see Fear of Annihilation, Section 7). Sometimes there are more tangible reasons for the child's fear of the bath, such as the water being too hot or a past experience of slipping in the tub.

This fear cannot be forcibly overcome. The best thing is to wash the child outside the bathtub for a while. Then reacquaint him with the pleasure of bathing by allowing him to splash with his hands, and only gradually put him in a tub with very little water.

SECTION 9. *Fear of Bedwetting*

Toilet training is usually completed in the fourth year of life. Some children are completely trained toward the end of the third year, but many need one year or so more.

CHILDREN'S FEARS

If a three-and-a-half-year-old fails to control his bladder, he may be a latecomer, but there is nothing to worry about.

Bedwetting is a problem in older children who have never attained bladder control or have lost self-control and regressed to an earlier level of development.

Epileptic children, children with abnormalities of the spinal cord, or those suffering kidney or bladder infection must be excluded at this point; their difficulties with bladder control require medical attention.

Some girls who fear sex try to outdo males, and act as if they were boys. One of the clear differences between the sexes is the manner in which they urinate. Little boys often show off with their ability to piss high and far, and this makes them feel high and mighty. A girl worried about her fear of sex or lack of success with men may develop the desire to act like a boy and unconsciously wish to urinate like one. She will control her wish during her waking hours, but at night she may dream that she urinates like a boy—and her dream comes true, to her own embarrassment and her mother's dismay.

Some boys who are bedwetters are motivated by a similar dynamism. Usually they are children of aggressive, domineering women, and they tend to accept a passive and submissive role. They seem not to accept much responsibility for what happens to them, and in sleep they "let things flow."

When a bedwetter is punished, this does not stop the bedwetting but rather makes the child afraid to fall asleep.

Bedwetting comes to an end in practically all cases at the onset of puberty. If it is excessive, the child may need psychological help, but in most cases, the less attention paid to it, and the more reassurance given to the child, the sooner it will end.

CHILDREN'S FEARS IN ALPHABETICAL ORDER

SECTION 10. *Fear of Being an Adopted Child*

This fear is most frequent in school-age children. One study discovered that 28 percent of children between the ages of eight and twelve feared that their parents were not their real parents but had adopted them. It is worthwhile mentioning that only 6 percent of the mothers reported in that study were aware of their children's fear of being adopted.

The origin of this imaginary fear lies in overt or covert parental rejection. When parents display impatience and irritability, when they often and harshly punish the child, the child may develop the frightening fantasy that they are not his real parents.

SECTION 11. *Fear of Change*

Moving, traveling, and meeting new people can be either enjoyable or frightening, depending on the child's developmental phase and parental attitudes.

Adults welcome a change, provided it brings enjoyment. Most people like pleasant surprises, exciting trips, and new and friendly acquaintances. Curiosity and the need for change are universal human traits, but even adults may hesitate to plunge into a totally new and unpredictable situation.

Certainly no human being welcomes a change for the worse. Wise parents know that while moving to larger quarters in a better environment is enjoyable to them, it is not necessarily a pleasure to their small child. For him, the new house represents the unfamiliar and the unknown and could therefore be threatening.

A little child derives security from *continuity*. He knows what and whom to expect at his crib or bed every morning. He knows where the kitchen is and how to find his toys. Continuity of daily life, the *sameness* of people and things around him, builds his feeling of safety.

Because the new house that is a source of pride and joy to his parents may be frightening to a two- or three-year-old, he needs a good deal of protective guidance. The parents should take him around the new house, and show him that his favorite high chair, bed, and toys have made the move with him.

Traveling with a two-year-old may be trying because children this age show no enthusiasm for Versailles or appreciation for the art collections in Rome. They prefer their own corner at home and do not share their parents' curiosity about European architecture. Should travel be necessary, the parents should bring along something old to reassure the child.

Should it be necessary to hire a housekeeper, a cleaning person, or a new babysitter, the intruder (as the child views her) should be introduced gradually. The new person should not be left alone with the child until he has had the chance to get used to her.

In *The Widening World of Childhood,* p. 101, Dr. Lois B. Murphy described how a mother handled her three-year-old daughter. When the little girl was told they were moving, she said, "I'm not going to move." The mother explained that the father had to go to a new job, and added, "I'm going and Billy is going and Trudy's going and our dog is going and the cat is going, and you can take your furniture and your teddy bear, and you can have all your things in your new room and in the new house." The little girl agreed to go.

SECTION 12. *Fear of Castration*

Castration fear usually starts at the age of three to five, during the period called *phallic* by Sigmund Freud. At this time boys experience the so-called Oedipus complex, named for the King of Thebes who killed his father and married his mother. Oedipus's tragedy was not a result of malevolence on his part, but a product of inevitable fate. When he realized what he had done, however, he punished himself by putting out his eyes. Freud saw in this myth a symbolic description of the prehistoric development of human society and, in accordance with the biogenetic principle, a necessary stage in the lives of individuals. Freud discovered that every three to five year-old boy desires to possess his mother physically in the ways he has learned from observation and intuitive surmises of sexual life, and tries to seduce her by showing her the male organ of which he is the proud owner. The boy wants to take his father's place, for although he loves and admires his father, at the same time he views him as a competitor and wishes to get rid of him (see Chapter V).

To explain the boy's ambivalent feelings toward his father, and the girl's ambivalent feelings toward her mother, Freud assumed that everyone is inherently bisexual. Each sex is attracted to members of the same sex as well as to members of the opposite sex. Freud felt this to be the constitutional basis for homosexuality, although in most people the homosexual impulses remain latent.

Bisexuality complicates the Oedipus complex by inducing sexual cathexes for the same-sex parent, so that the boy's feelings for his father and the girl's for her mother are said to be ambivalent, rather than univalent, in character. This assumption of bisexuality has recently been supported by investigations on the endocrine glands that show rather conclusively that both male and female sex hormones are present in each sex.

To return to the description of the phallic phase, at this time the penis becomes the main source of pleasurable

CHILDREN'S FEARS

sensations in the boy. In contradistinction to the more passive and earlier desire to be fondled, a definite wish emerges for active pursuit and thrust with the penis. However, the little boy is aware of his inferiority in comparison to his father, whose penis is larger. He is afraid that his father will punish him for masturbation and for desiring his mother. If the boy has previously noticed the difference between male and female organs, the threat of castration becomes something very realistic and shocking. He may believe that originally all people have a penis but that it is sometimes cut off by an omnipotent father. This fear of castration is much stronger than the oral fear of being eaten or the anal fear of losing the body content.

In normal child development the conflict resolves itself in due course.

SECTION 13. *Fear of Cripples*

Preschool children tend to project and identify with others. The sight of a cripple may make them worry about themselves and fear that they too may become crippled.

Usually simple reassurance will suffice. After all, most crippled people adjust to life, hold jobs, and lead normal family lives. After a war, when children encounter many crippled veterans, parents should elicit respect for the veterans' courage and devotion and instill in the child the feeling of solidarity with his own people. (This was the advice I gave to my colleagues in Israel after the October 1973 war.)

SECTION 14. *Fear of Criticism*

No one likes to be criticized, but children are likely to perceive criticism as rejection. Sensitive, shy, and anxious children may blame themselves for mild or uncommitted sins.

Parents should avoid overgeneralized negative criti-

cism such as "You are careless, you *always* break cups."
Positive criticism may help the child, such as "When you
carry the cup, please hold on to the saucer and the cup.
This way we avoid trouble."

Ridicule is another form of criticism (see Section 36).

SECTION 15. *Fear of Darkness*

In darkness one is less capable of noticing dangers
and less in touch with potential allies. In darkness one's
own power is reduced, the readiness to defend oneself is
impaired, and the chances for obtaining help are di-
minished. In darkness fears—of the unfamiliar and of
loneliness—are combined.

Although the fear of the unfamiliar is described in
Section 46 and the fear of loneliness in Section 29, the fear
of darkness deserves a more detailed analysis. It is rooted
in childhood and never completely disappears, but it as-
sumes various forms and is acted upon in different ways in
different circumstances. Of course, one does not fear
darkness when in a familiar and well-protected environment surrounded by trustworthy people. But even mature
adults prefer lighted streets to dark ones, a safe environment to an unsafe one, and friendly companions to loneliness or strangers.

A child's physical and mental equipment are small
protection, and even in full light he or she will fear the
unfamiliar and strange and get panicky when lost and
lonely. The child's natural makeup does not prepare him
to face hardships, and unless protected by loving parents
or a parental substitute, he may not survive. While his
physical survival depends on the supply of food, shelter,
and physical protection, his mental well-being depends on
how all these things are furnished. Harry Stack Sullivan
observed that early childhood experiences play a very im-

portant role in the development of a person's feeling of security. The infant knows by empathy whether or not he is accepted, and a loved child develops a feeling of well-being and happiness. This is the feeling of euphoria. The need for satisfaction and the need for security follow the same path. The same mother feeds and cuddles, the same feeding process serves satisfaction and security.

In *Conceptions of Modern Psychiatry*, p. 7, Sullivan wrote that from the very first days of life, "the infant shows a curious relationship or connection with the significant adult, ordinarily the mother. If the mother . . . is seriously disturbed . . . around the time of feeding, then on that occasion there will be feeding difficulty or the infant will have indigestion." A child who feels lonely and unloved may develop profound anxiety states.

It is easy for an adult who has developed adequate knowledge of his close environment and has good motor coordination to move around in a dark or poorly lit room, especially when he feels safe. But a child does not have this knowledge or coordination, and in the darkness an armchair may look like a horror figure he saw on television. As he tries to please his parents and moves slowly about the dark room, he may stumble over the vicious carpet or bang against the mean lamp, hurt himself, and consequently fear darkness even more.

In darkness familiar things look unfamiliar. Preschool children's imagination leads them to ascribe human traits to inanimate objects and makes them believe that pieces of furniture or other objects can get nasty. Sometimes children project their own hostile wishes on pets or inanimate objects, and then become afraid of the figments of their own imagination. Darkness reduces contact with the real world, gives vent to the imagination, and creates the feeling of loneliness.

Feeling lonely and forsaken is the main cause of children's fears of darkness. Hardly anything is more frightening to a child than getting lost on a street or in a department store (See Chapter IV, V, and VI; and Sections 3, 29, and 37). The fear of being lost or abandoned has great survival value, for what indeed can a small child do for himself? Certainly every child must be encouraged to strive on his own, and *the road from birth to adulthood leads from a total dependence on others to a maximum of self-reliance. But this is a long and steep uphill road, and children need not be forced to run before they are ready to walk.*

A child needs adult support. As the child grows wiser and stronger, the support gradually decreases. To force a frightened child to be alone in a dark room is an unnecessary and unwarranted effort to break the laws of natural development. Most children feel lonely in darkness. They cannot see their parents and their familiar surroundings, and to punish them for "being chicken" or "babies" is tantamount to punishing a blind man because he does not see.

A small night light in the child's bedroom will not spoil him, it will merely help him outgrow the fear of darkness. Neither he nor his parents will ever completely outgrow their fear of darkness and its two major components, the fear of loneliness and the fear of the unfamiliar, but the fear will gradually diminish to rational dimensions.

SECTION 16. *Fear of Death*

All human beings (and all other living creatures) fear death, but most people who lead an active and satisfactory life are not preoccupied with this idea. Fear of death is activated by the potential proximity of death, such as severe illness, injury, or the threat of either.

Almost every child experiences the fear of death in the difficult moments of his life. In some children this fear is aroused by a death in the family, in others by their own sickness or other traumatic events.

A child's fear of death signals his profound feelings of helplessness, loneliness, and hopelessness. Under favorable circumstances the child gradually feels stronger as he grows, and takes pride in his increasing size, muscular strength, motor agility, and so on. Children need continual parental confirmation of their growth. "My, you are so big," a smart mother says, and the little girl may add, "Do you remember when I was little and I could not do this?" A brief and reassuring explanation and pleasant activities help the child and allay his worries.

SECTION 17. *Fear of Disapproval and Rejection*

Many children fear parental disapproval and rejection. Of course, parents must occasionally express disapproval of the child's behavior. They must, however, stress that they disapprove of a particular action. They may sternly say, "I don't like what you have done. You must not do it again." They must not say, "I don't like you. You are a bad child."

A child who feels rejected may develop a profound and pervading feeling of anxiety that may affect his future social adjustment. The need to be accepted by others is universal and all human beings like to be liked. The intensity of this need greatly depends on early childhood experiences, and an overdependence on being accepted by others may adversely affect one's social adjustment.

A child who feels accepted and loved by his parents is likely to develop an air of assuredness that wins friends. As explained in Chapter I, people tend to associate with those they perceive as self-assured (strong) and friendly. One who grew up in a congenial home atmosphere enters the world of peers and adults with the feeling of being accepted, and he is willing to reciprocate. Of course, he may suffer social setbacks, be rejected and hurt, but he is reasonably well prepared to face these inevitable hardships and frustrations.

A child who feels rejected by his parents enters the world with the fear that no one will like him. If his own parents don't care for him, who will? The less he hopes for acceptance, the more he craves it, and this attitude is a self-fulfilling prophesy. An insecure, frightened child will hardly attract friends because his fear of being rejected makes him shy away from people, although he craves their company and approval. He wishes to make friends but he fears to reach out. He gives the impression of being both weak and hostile, and his clumsy social behavior invites ridicule and ostracism, which in turn make him even more frightened and withdrawn.

A child who fears peer rejection, and whose behavior unwillingly and unwittingly increases the chances for such a rejection, needs a lot of parental support. Unfortunately some parents blame the child for being unpopular and thus make him feel even more lonely and insecure. Some even side with their child's adversaries, as if to say (and sometimes do say blatantly) "Nobody likes you because you are weak, a coward, stupid," and so on.

If a frightened child receives reassurance, his self-esteem will improve and he will become less dependent on outside approval, less tense, and less vulnerable—all of which will improve his chances for good social relations.

Outright rejection by peers and/or teachers requires consultation with the school psychologist or guidance worker.

SECTION 18. *Fear of Divorce*

An eight-year-old girl was reported as having a severe school phobia. She refused to go to school, and when her parents tried to force her, she threw up. Her sleep was highly disturbed and full of nightmares. The reason she gave for her fear of going to school did not make any sense: she told her parents that the teacher had scolded another child and was generally irritable.

Actually she had overheard her parents' arguments and knew they had decided to separate. Late at night, on the eve of the onset of her phobia, her parents discussed their decision, unaware that their eight-year-old daughter was lying awake in bed listening to them. The little girl knew she was supposed to be asleep. That morning her mother told her that her father was "temporarily" moving out. "He will come home from work early today and pack his belongings."

All children dread divorce and there are no foolproof methods for allaying this fear. It is better not to fan this fear by unnecessary and premature talk. When breaking up is certain or imminent, children should be told and assured that *both* parents love them, and one of the parents will see them on certain days.

SECTION 19. *Fear of Failure*

The desire to be successful is a universal human trait not related to age, sex, or cultural background. Achievement is the natural reward for effort. The greater the effort, the greater is the expectancy of achievement.

People enjoy many things, such as food, sex, and leisure, but only great achievements, victories, and triumphs make one really happy. Happiness is a winged creature; it comes at moments of great success and goes away waiting for new and fresh victories.

In childhood success usually brings parental praise. A child's estimate of his achievements is greatly influenced by his parents' attitude. His self-esteem is determined by their approval, and every child desperately needs to hear that he or she is nice, good, smart, and so on.

Everyone learns pretty soon in life that nobody can expect to be successful always and in everything. We learn to accept failure and defeat as inescapable, but the setbacks need not discourage future efforts nor damage our self-esteem. The child must learn that rational self-esteem derives from a realistic appraisal of what one is supposed to do and what one can do. The development of such inner balance greatly depends on parental attitudes.

Parents should make demands, for the acceptance of parental rules, admonitions, and prohibitions helps the child to develop his own self-discipline and moral code. Parents who are too lenient do not help their child in his growth and maturation. Parents who approve of whatever the child does distort his sense of reality and foster a selfish, inconsiderate personality.

However, parents must not become too demanding, harsh, and rejecting. A child needs a reasonable amount of praise when he is successful, and a reasonable amount of reassurance and encouragement when he fails. Parents should give credit for efforts such as the child's help in washing dishes, even if he breaks a cup. Of course, there is no reason to praise laziness, sloppiness, and disobedience, but there is no reason to blame a child for mishap or failure, especially if it is beyond his control or the task was unreasonably difficult.

Parents who expect too much and too early produce an overt fear of failure and an unconscious state of anxiety in their children. Some become so afraid of failing and of being criticized that they develop severe withdrawal symptoms and acute anxiety, which require professional help.

SECTION 20.   *Fear of Fairy Tales*

Many fairy tales are folkloristic allusions to human frailty, greed, and aggressiveness. Some of them involve mean witches, cruel kings, greedy wolves, and other scary characters.

Preschool children and young school-age children often confuse make-believe with reality. They may fear that the horrible witch will come and snatch them, or put them to sleep for one hundred years, or play some other dirty trick on them. Of course, not all children are scared by fairy tales, but more sensitive, anxious children should be spared the horrifying stories.

The *sight* of horror has a much stronger and worse effect on children; many television programs produce great fear and anxiety in preschool and grade-school children.

SECTION 21.   *Fear of Food*

Anxious mothers may evoke fear of certain types of food as early as the first or second year of life. Normally nature regulates infants' appetites and tastes, and wise mothers know their infants' whims and preferences. Should a mother insist on feeding the infant when he is in no mood for a meal, or demand he finish a particular dish he dislikes, she may create quite a problem. The infant becomes afraid of her feeding methods, and his fear of one particular dish may spread until it seriously disturbs all his eating habits. He may develop nausea, gagging, and other eating difficulties.

Too radical a weaning from breast or bottle, and forcing the infant to eat solid food before he is ready for it, may cause fears of choking and vomiting.

The best way to overcome the fear of food is to feed

the child his favorite dishes in quantities he likes, and allow him to eat only when he is hungry.

SECTION 22. *Fear of Future Dangers*

The child's ability to anticipate the consequences of his or her actions is rather limited. Even adolescents have a rather limited ability to predict the outcome of their deeds, and they often take unnecessary and harmful risks because they gravely underestimate the potential dangers.

When a five- or six- or seven-year-old expresses apprehension not related to present or imminent danger but to some unpredictable future event, his emotion is probably anxiety rather than fear. (Anxiety is described in Section 2.)

SECTION 23. *Fear and Guilt*

Guilt is self-imposed punishment. This feeling may be either rational or irrational. It is irrational when a child feels that he is to blame for whatever misfortunes happen to himself, his parents, or other members of his family.

Parental admonitions may fan this guilt feeling. Parents warn their children, and rightly so, against taking unnecessary risks such as going out in the rain, being inadequately dressed in cold weather, and so on. Should a child catch a bad cold or break a leg, he may rightly feel it was his own fault.

Handicapped children sometimes blame themselves for their handicap, even if it is congenital or the result of an uncontrollable disease. I have had in psychological treatment victims of polio who blamed themselves for being sick, and felt guilty for all the pain they caused their parents.

Guilt feelings may make one wish to be punished and fear the seemingly unavoidable punishment. Children (and adults) torn by guilt may become prophets of gloom,

CHILDREN'S FEARS

and their potential misfortunes nothing but self-fulfilling prophesies. Their unconscious wish to be punished can bring disaster upon them. Sometimes children who blame themselves for misfortunes they did not cause provoke their parents, unconsciously wishing to be severely punished. Their fear of feeling guilty makes them bring upon themselves the punishment they fear and wish for at the same time.

It is normal for a child to feel guilty when he does something wrong, but parents must avoid creating *unnecessary* guilt feelings in their child by blaming him for sins he did not commit. When a mother breaks a dish because *she* was careless, she must not tell the child, "It's all because of you."

It is interesting to watch mothers whose children play in a sandbox or with mud. When the child smears his face, his shirt, and everything else, a smart mother will pick him up, smile, and wash him. An irrational mother will punish him unjustly. But worse is the mother who says, "All right, get yourself dirty. I spent a lot of time washing and ironing your clothes. Now I know that you don't love your mother."

SECTION 24. *Fear of Homosexuality*

Many preadolescent and adolescent boys and girls fear that they may become homosexuals. Preadolescents tend to form close friendships with a person of the same sex, and preadolescent crushes on a person of the same sex are common occurrences.

As a rule, the less attention paid, the better; but serious cases of homosexual panic require professional help (see Section 38).

CHILDREN'S FEARS IN ALPHABETICAL ORDER

SECTION 25. *Fear of Hospitalization*

There must be a very serious health reason for putting an infant in the hospital, for such a forced separation from parents and home environment is likely to elicit grave fear reactions.

Dr. John Bowlby, in his book *Attachment and Loss,* has described the emotional reactions of hospitalized toddlers. Their initial reaction is vehement: they cry, scream, bang their heads, and fight anyone who tries to take care of them.

After a few hours or a day or two of violent kicking and screaming, the infant seems to give up all hope. He may whine or whimper, but he will allow hospital personnel to do as they please without offering any resistance.

In the third phase the infant seems to have accepted the new situation and responds to friendly overtures from the hospital staff. His emotional reactions are shallow, however, and he seems to be uninvolved with anyone, even his own parents when they visit him.

In order to prevent these unhealthy fear reactions the mother should stay in the hospital with her infant and let him bring from home his favorite toys.

SECTION 26. *Fear of Injury*

Fear of being hurt or injured is common to all human beings. This fear should not be discouraged. A child should be taught to take necessary precautions when walking on ice, swimming, and so on.

The fear must not be aggravated by exaggerated parental reaction. Prompt and matter-of-fact attention reduces fear and contributes to the child's feeling of security.

SECTION 27. *Fear of Insects*

It may seem strange that a child who safely plays with a huge pet dog is frightened by a tiny crawling ant or a buzzing mosquito. The fear of insects is often associated with fear of the unknown, the unpredictable, and familiarity with insects will help the child to overcome his fears.

A child who squashes an insect may develop a fear of revenge by the insect's family or friends. Such a fear may be indicative of other fears, perhaps of the child's fear of his own aggressivity (see Section 5).

SECTION 28. *Fear of Lack of Food*

When a hungry infant is not given food he may fear that no food will ever be given to him. This is a frightening and unhealthy feeling. The child who worries about getting food may later in life tend to overeat. He may also become excessively demanding and greedy.

Later in life he may worry unrealistically about business failure, poverty, depression, and famine. Sometimes this fear spreads so that he is scared he'll never get enough love and recognition. He may become envious of everyone else and assume that everyone is better off than he is.

SECTION 29. *Fear of Being Alone*

Even adults sometimes fear being alone, but practically all children have this fear. The younger the child, the greater the fear. The physical presence of someone perceived as strong and friendly substantially reduces it. Just the sight of the mother or the father has a calming effect on a scared child.

SECTION 30. *Fear of Loss of Balance*

Loss of balance, stumbling, and falling are universally feared by young and old alike. It is apparently innate, for even newborns and children a few days old cry and startle when they lose support.

There is no way (nor reason) to overcome this fear. The fear of loss of balance has survival value, for it makes one cautious when leaning out of a window, climbing mountains, and walking on icy surfaces. Fearless individuals may pay a high price for their recklessness, and wise parents do not encourage brazen and foolhardy behavior. Newton's law of gravity certainly deserves respect from people who choose to stay alive!

There is good reason, of course, to prevent exaggerated and unrealistic fears, such as the fear of climbing stairs, being near an open window, or going out on a cold day. Sometimes such a fear is not genuine but *displaced,* serving as a cover-up for another fear or anxiety.

Normally, as the child grows older, his motor coordination improves and this fear gradually diminishes.

SECTION 31. *Fear of Loss of Love*

Child psychologists and psychiatrists have noticed that *milk is not enough.* Infants must feel that the milk that is given to them is a sign of love and affection.

The fear of loss of parental love is terrifying to an infant and even an older child. Parents may, when necessary, scold a child or punish him, but they should never threaten to withdraw their love.

SECTION 32. *Fear of Noise*

The fear of loud and sudden noise is innate. Newborn babies when they hear a sudden and loud noise react automatically with apparent signs of fright.

There is no way to prevent this reaction to loud and sudden noises. Many birds and animals use loud noise as an alarm signal, and a sharp, loud call—"Watch out!"—is a standard human warning signal. Sharp, sudden sounds put human beings on alert and enable them to mobilize their resources for fight or flight. An explosion induces everyone to run for his life, and in time of war the wailing of sirens makes people rush to air raid shelters.

While loud, sudden, and unexpected sounds produce a startle and fear reaction at all ages, there is a gradual elimination of fear reaction to certain loud noises, and an acquisition of sensitivity to other sounds. For instance, if the father is a cabinetmaker who works at home, the child will get used to heavy banging.

In the first year of life the infant is frightened by very loud and sudden noises, but may not react to the buzzing of a bee or the hissing of a cat. An older child, more aware of the potential danger, is frightened by the latter noises.

SECTION 33. *Fear of Parents*

In normal circumstances the child perceives his parents as being both strong (capable of protecting him and taking care of him) and *friendly* (willing to do so). The child's fears therefore can take two directions: He may fear that his parents will lose their strength and become *unable* to take care of him, or he may be afraid that they become unfriendly and thus *unwilling* to take care of him. In the first case the child worries about his parents and may blame himself for their real or imaginary sickness and other misfortunes. In the second he may feel unworthy and undeserving of parental love.

Either fear may produce severe anxiety (see Section 2), but a certain degree of the second type of fear is necessary for normal development. People abstain from antisocial behavior for two reasons: *restraint from without* and/or *self-restraint.* Restraint from without is tantamount to fear of retaliation and punishment, and if parents intend to bring their child up rationally, they must set limits to his freedom and establish definite rules.

People who feel that they can get away with murder are more inclined to murder than people who fear the consequences of their antisocial behavior. If parents condone antisocial acts and dishonesty, and/or themselves set such an example, the child is likely to develop an antisocial personality.

Rational child rearing employs both love and fear. Children need to be loved and taken care of, but they must also learn to fear doing wrong if they are to become well-adjusted adults. The fear of parental disapproval and punishment is the first and necessary prerequisite for social adjustment.

Well-adjusted and honest adults do not act on impulse and do not hurt other people mainly because they have developed *inner inhibitions* and *self-control*. A human infant comes into the world without any inhibitions whatsoever. Infants urinate and eliminate the minute they feel pressure in the bladder or bowels; they cry when hurt, fall asleep when tired. They are self-centered and it takes years of growth before they develop consideration for others.

Parental love elicits the infant's love. The more loving and the more decisive, protective, and strong parents appear to the child, the more he is inclined to accept their rules and regulations. He loves them and fears losing their love. He incorporates their prohibitions and admonitions, and begins to act as if they were his own rules that he must obey. He identifies with his parents and develops a self-controlling and self-monitoring part of his personality, called by Freud the *superego*. The superego is the self-imposed control, the *conscience*, and represents the moral standards of his parents and society-at-large.

Parental love and fear of losing their love are the necessary ingredients of moral development.

SECTION 34. *Fear of Power Motors*

Many generations ago quick-moving, powerful beasts of prey represented a great danger to human lives. Today one is rarely exposed to ferocious beasts, but powerful household motors are a considerable danger to children. Wise parents caution their child not to touch electric outlets and switches of washing machines, dishwashers, dryers, vacuum cleaners, and so on.

Some parents, in an excess of caution, threaten the child with all kinds of potential catastrophes should he go near a busy washing machine or vacuum cleaner. The child's fantasy can go haywire. He may ascribe malicious thoughts to the washing machine that mercilessly hits his clothes, or be scared of the aggressive and greedy vacuum cleaner that swallows everything in its way.

Parents should neither underplay nor overplay potential dangers. Rather they should teach their child to take a rational middle road between careless and thoughtless risks on one side and paralyzing panic on the other (see Section 49).

SECTION 35. *Fear of Punishment*

The task of education is to help children become mature and well-adjusted adults, and responsibility for one's own actions is probably the main aspect of maturity. Human behavior is a chain of causes and effects, and mature individuals assume full responsibility for their deeds. They are aware of the consequences of their actions, and know that these consequences can be quite painful. This realistic awareness is a prerequisite for adjustment to other people and to life in general.

It is necessary to convey to children this cause-and-ef-

CHILDREN'S FEARS IN ALPHABETICAL ORDER

fect lesson. As with any other lesson, it must not start too early or too harshly; it must be introduced gradually. It is better that the child be *told* the consequences of his behavior than be allowed to make mistakes and then be punished for them. It is always better to *prevent* misbehavior than to punish it.

Should parents feel that, in a particular case, punishment is the right method, they should try to be as calm and rational about it as possible. A screaming, livid parent may evoke fear and hatred instead of repentance. Punishment should be reasonable, in proportion to the transgression, and, most importantly, close the issue. "You did not prepare your homework, and you will be deprived of TV for a certain period" is sufficient. Do not bring the incident up again and again. Punishment should never take the form of a withdrawal of love. Parents must often disapprove of their child's behavior, but they should never disapprove of their child or reject him (see Sections 3, 17, and 33).

Parents who indulge in frequent and harsh punishment are likely to be disappointed in the results of their method. If they are inconsistent in their policy, the child will perceive them as being weak and hostile, and soon disrespect them. If their harsh and punitive policy is consistent, the child will perceive them as strong and hostile, and develop a fear of and hatred toward them. Excessive fear of punishment may play havoc with the child's personality. He may identify with the punitive parents and act in an aggressive, hostile manner toward smaller and weaker children, and his adult behavior may be influenced by the treatment he experienced as a helpless child.

Punishment can be useful if it is rare and fair, and when the child understands that it is justified and meant for his well-being. Parental temper tantrums can harm a child's future adjustment.

SECTION 36. *Fear of Ridicule*

Small infants do not react to ridicule because they do not comprehend it, but older children are far more sensitive to it.

Ridicule is a psychological assault that makes the victim feel small, weak, inadequate, and stupid. The ridiculing person derives a good deal of pleasure from this self-aggrandizement at the expense of someone who is usually unable to retaliate. Parents and teachers must not use this method, for it is both cruel and counterproductive. A child who fears ridicule may refrain from many useful and enjoyable activities such as sports, music, and drawing. Fear of being ridiculed undermines self-esteem and self-confidence.

School-age children quite often ridicule another child chosen to be the target of their hostile behavior because he is smaller or weaker, a member of a minority group, a lonely child, or anyone unable to retaliate. Adults should intervene and explain to those who ridicule that this is hostile and unfair self-aggrandizement.

SECTION 37. *Fear of Separation*

One of the most frequent childhood fears is the fear of separation from the parents, especially the mother. Separation anxiety is a genuine fear reaction and, basically, a normal and useful emotion. A little child cannot survive unless someone takes care of him, and the loss of a caring person represents a most serious threat. An infant who dares to wander away from his mother may run into great trouble, so he is better off if he is afraid of getting lost. When a two- or three-year-old goes shopping with his mother, it is with good reason that he holds onto her for dear life.

CHILDREN'S FEARS IN ALPHABETICAL ORDER

This emotional reaction may outlive its usefulness, however. Older children must learn to become more self-reliant and independent. Becoming independent is a gradual process, and every child must be allowed to proceed according to his abilities. Parents should not push a timid child to attain the level of independence the neighbor's aggressive child has attained, but they must not prevent this process of maturation by overprotection.

In most cases (but by all means not all) the fear of separation starts in the second half of the first year of life. In the first six or seven months infants indiscriminately respond to whoever takes care of them. Most probably they need this time to get acquainted with their environment.

Around the twenty-eighth week of life most infants develop a fear of strangers. Apparently they have learned to distinguish between familiar and unfamiliar faces, and armed with this new talent, they begin to be choosy. They certainly prefer to stay with those they know and trust and to avoid unknown and unfamiliar faces and situations (see Section 46). They hold onto mother, father, grandmother, and other familiar people, and cry in fear when mother goes away and leaves them with a strange babysitter.

This fear of separation can be aggravated or ameliorated by parental attitudes and actions. If parents isolate the child so that he spends all his time in their company, sleeps in their room, is not allowed to play with other children, and has no visitors, the infant will certainly become overattached to them and panic at their absence. Isolation will unnecessarily aggravate and perpetuate the fear of separation.

Of course, socialization of the child should proceed consistently and gradually. There is a limit to the infant's ability to relate to other people, and there is no reason to overtax it by exposing him in the first two years of his life to an army of relatives and acquaintances. Relatives and friends should be introduced gradually, piecemeal as it were. It is good to have grandparents or uncles and aunts pay frequent visits, stay a while, and play with the infant. The infant will learn to feel at ease with them and thus enlarge his social contacts. A new babysitter should not be left alone with the baby at first. The mother should stay with the babysitter and the child for a while, and leave only when she is sure the infant feels happy with the babysitter.

Parental attitudes are often communicated nonverbally to the infant. When the mother dislikes her mother-in-law, the infant may share her feelings. When the mother likes the new housekeeper and is overtly friendly toward her, the chances are that the infant won't mind his mother's absence.

An early and too prolonged separation is likely to be quite disturbing to children. During the London Blitz in the Second World War many children were evacuated and sent to much safer rural areas. There is adequate evidence that those who were separated from their parents were more disturbed than those who stayed with their parents in London under heavy air bombardment.

Infants below twenty weeks of age show little reaction when separated from their mothers, admitted to a hospital, or placed away from their parents. At the age of twenty-eight weeks, however, they become restless, cry, struggle, and suffer loss of appetite and sleep disturbance.

There is not much change in separation fears in the second and third year, although as the child learns that mother will indeed return, his fear gradually diminishes.

Generally the third year of life brings with it new separation fears, for children at this age are capable of anticipatory fears (younger children don't have the cognitive-anticipatory competence). A two-year-old is likely to be as upset as a one-year-old at a separation, but a three-year-old may be more upset, unless he is absolutely certain his mother will come back at a promised time—and children seem to have built-in clocks.

In the third and fourth year of life most children are fearful their first day in a nursery. Their emotional reaction depends on past experience. Those who are sure that mother keeps her promises and always shows up at the agreed upon time accept separation with less anxiety. Children who distrust their mothers anxiously cling to them.

At the age of five or six less than 25 percent of children have intense separation fears their first day in school. The frequency and intensity of their fears is determined by their trust or mistrust of their parents and by the amount of social exposure they have had at home, in the playground, and elsewhere.

Should the fear of separation persist into the school years, it might represent an ambivalent attitude toward the parents. The child who harbors hostile feelings toward one or both of them needs their physical presence for reassurance that his aggressive fantasies and destructive wishes have not come true.

Separation fear is also perpetuated by parental over-protection and *their* need for the child's physical presence. Clinging parents invite separation fear, and quite often a child who feels his parents need him feels guilty and frightened when away from home. School phobia is often produced by such an inappropriate parental attitude (see Section 52).

SECTION 38. *Fear of Sex*

Fear of sexual encounters looms large among the

CHILDREN'S FEARS

fears of preadolescent and adolescent boys and girls. In boys this fear is usually related to self-confidence and psychosexual identification. Some boys feel that their penises are small or that they will never perform well sexually or that they are not too manly in general.

The popular and oversimplified notion of manliness stresses physical size, muscular strength, courage, decisiveness, enterprising spirit, and sexual prowess. Unfortunately this somewhat archaic notion is supported by the mass media, in which supermen, gangsters, and hoodlums are presented as models of masculinity, despite the fact that most of the great men in history have been hardworking, wise, and responsible.

Peer groups foster machismo. Youngsters who brag often become leaders of the gang, while shy and timid boys are ridiculed. Many girls are attracted by displays of power. Flattered by the attention of boisterous gang leaders, this type of girl looks down on boys who are not outspoken and self-assertive.

The less courage an adolescent boy displays, the fewer his chances with girls. Fear of sexual relations is most often associated with an overall feeling of weakness and inadequacy. A boy who thinks little of himself may fear girls' rejection. This fear becomes a self-fulfilling prophesy—the less he thinks of himself, the less able he is to attract girls. It is a vicious circle: Insecure boys develop a profound fear of sexual intercourse and then perform poorly as lovers. Though they may believe their penises are too small or their erection is inadequate, their frustration and failure in sexual encounters are self-induced.

Girls' sexual fears are usually related to physical appearance, or actually, to what a girl thinks of her own appearance. I have had in psychotherapeutic treatment attractive girls who described themselves as ugly ducklings.

CHILDREN'S FEARS IN ALPHABETICAL ORDER

The reasons for such low self-esteem varied, but whenever their body-image was unfavorable, they feared boys, sexual foreplay, and sexual relations. They felt unattractive and expected rejection—an attitude that turned into a self-fulfilling prophesy. One of my adolescent patients maintained that no boy would ever take her out or make advances to her. She knew for sure that she could never satisfy a man and avoided male company out of fear of failure.

Many sexual fears are rooted in the early years, especially from three to six. Most children undergo at this age what Sigmund Freud called the "family romance" or "Oedipus complex." Preschool children tend to develop a sexual attachment to the parent of the opposite sex, and view the parent of the same sex as an intruder and competitor. This love-hate for the parent of the same sex and great love for the parent of the opposite sex is gradually resolved in later years through identification with the parent of the same sex. Inadequate psychosexual identification in childhood may be one of the main causes of disturbances in sexual behavior in adulthood (see Chapters V and VII).

Sexual fears are often linked to general personality difficulties and in most cases they call for professional help (see also Sections 12 and 24).

SECTION 39. *Fear of Showing Fear*

Some parents expect their child to be brave and understanding. They seem to believe that telling the child there are no spooks, or that injections do not hurt, will convince the little boy or girl. Fear of parental disapproval or ridicule may make the child hide his fears and pretend that he is unafraid of darkness, doctors, dentists, and big dogs. Sometimes the original fear becomes displaced by another fear that is less embarrassing and less likely to be criticized by parents (See Section 51, Phobias).

A child who believes he must hide his fears very often becomes even more frightened and unhappy. He or she may get into real trouble by pretending to be brave.

It is advisable to allow a child to express his fears and deal with them in a rational way, as described in Chapter VIII.

SECTION 40. *Fear of Sleep*

The fear of falling asleep usually develops in the second year of life. The same infant who used to fall asleep at the drop of a hat, who dozed off whenever satiated, tired, or just comfortable, a few months later may refuse to go to sleep, even when very tired. He may toss and turn in his crib, ask innumerable questions, cry, call for his mother, demand that the door be open, ask for a drink of water, and put his parents' patience to the test.

At this age infants have already developed emotional ties to their parents and they feel safe when they see the familiar faces and hear the familiar voices. To them, falling asleep means giving up the feeling of security and plunging into the unknown world of aloneness.

Parents should not punish a toddler who frets at bedtime, but neither should they reward him. They must be firm and friendly, neither giving in nor showing annoyance. They must understand that this difficulty will resolve itself as soon as the infant develops more faith in himself and feels more secure.

The refusal to sleep is related to the child's fear of abandonment. It is often designed to outsmart parents who put the small child to sleep and then go out and come home at ungodly hours. Because he does not trust them and fears they will leave him as soon as he falls asleep, the child may lie awake in bed listening to his parents' voices.

To make sure that they are still there, he may march into the living room with the sweetest smile and ask for just one sip of milk or water.

To help the child overcome the fear of falling asleep parents should build *self-confidence* by assuring the infant that he or she is big, nice, strong, and can fall asleep alone. At the same time, they must demonstrate that they love the child and will remain nearby. Self-confidence and the assurance of continued parental love are the best medicine for sleep disturbance.

Sometimes a child again experiences the fear of falling asleep at school age. He may fear imaginary supernatural forces (see Section 48); sometimes his own dreams and nightmares frighten him (see Section 50). In all these cases parental reaction should be neither punitive nor rewarding. Rather parents should help the child build self-confidence and faith in their love and protection. A strong person who has powerful and dependable allies need not fear.

Under no circumstances and at no age should parents add insult to injury by ridiculing or punishing a frightened child. Such a policy could result in increased fears. Nor should the parents yield to the child's demands, sit on his bed, or allow him to get into their bed. Such concessions reward the child's fears and perpetuate them.

SECTION 41. *Fear of Snakes*

Animals evoke in children ambivalent feelings of interest and fear. It seems that snakes are the most feared animals by children of almost all ages. A few years ago a British television network interviewed twelve thousand children, aged four and up, and found the snake was the most disliked and feared animal; spiders came next.

The fear of snakes is more related to parental attitudes than to the way snakes look and move. Adults have good reason to fear poisonous snakes that could attack them suddenly, out of nowhere, and they communicate this fear to their children, verbally or nonverbally. Since a child may not have adequate knowledge of the potential danger of snakes, this fear has a survival value.

SECTION 42. *Fear of Strangers*

At about six to ten months most infants develop fears of strangers. This fear is perfectly normal. The infant's mental development involves improved perception and memory. While he readily recognizes familiar household faces and expects food and affection from them, who can tell what a stranger is up to?

Obviously the fear of strangers has some survival value and should not be criticized or suppressed. Even adults should not naively trust everyone, and a rational dose of caution won't hurt anyone.

However, this fear must not outlive its usefulness nor become too extensive and irrational. Children of paranoid, frightened, and suspicious parents are likely to accept parental attitudes. Rational behavior strikes a balance between a frightened avoidance of social contacts and a naive belief that the world is a nursery full of well-wishing daddies and mommies.

As the infant reaches the second year of life he may venture into the unknown and explore. He may observe visitors, follow and watch them. The mother's presence is reassuring, especially if she relates in a friendly manner to the visitor.

Parental guidance and a reasonable amount of assuredness help in building the child's self-confidence and enable him to dare without becoming thoughtless and brazen (see Section 49 on lack of fear).

SECTION 43. *Fear of Subways*

A child who travels by subway on his mother's lap or sits next to his father rarely develops any particular fears about a subway ride. However, later in life some school-age children and adolescents who ride alone do develop such fears.

There is a realistic aspect to this fear because, unfortunately, a subway is not the safest place. Moreover, excluding the threats of muggers and hoodlums, the very fact of being alone, and having no way of anticipating motion, speed, and direction (as one has in a car or cab), may be conducive to some degree of insecurity.

This fear may be linked to a deep-seated anxiety. Anxious children fear change and try to control their environment. They may insist on certain daily routines that give them a feeling of control, for having control reduces the fear of the unpredictable. Being locked in a train over which they have no control may increase these children's anxiety.

Fear of subways is often a displaced fear or phobia (see Section 51). Sometimes it displaces the fear of not being able to prevent bad happenings at home. A child may worry that something bad will happen to his parents while he is locked into a subway car rushing to an unknown destination.

Although an exaggerated and unrealistic fear of subways often requires professional help, it could be substantially reduced and possibly resolved by a patient parent who for a while accompanies the frightened child on his rides.

SECTION 44. *Fear of Swimming*

Fear of deep water is well justified and no child should be forced into the water before he is able to cope with such an experience. Swimming lessons should be conducted in a safe environment with adequate supervision. As the child's swimming skill improves, his fear will gradually diminish.

A child's fear of water will increase if he is ridiculed or forcibly pushed into a swimming pool. The best way to handle this fear is to offer maximum protection, encouragement, and praise. An adult should go into the pool with the scared child, hold his hand, and wade with him in shallow waters. He or she should praise the child for wading so well, and encourage him to splash and to swim while offering support and protection.

SECTION 45. *Fear of Tests and Exams*

In any test or examination the examinee is judged and sentenced by the examiner. Teachers or the Board of Education arbitrarily prepare a set of questions they believe students should be able to answer. Those who do well on the test are rewarded by good marks, promotion to a higher grade, or admission to the desired school. Some degree of fear of tests should be expected and no child should be criticized for admitting this fear.

The examined student has no say in the choice of examiner, the questions he is expected to answer, or the examination procedures. Every school examination is likely to evoke (1) fear of the unknown; (2) fear of being punished and/or ridiculed; and (3) fear of being rejected.

The fear of a test or exam can have a beneficial effect if it stimulates effort. Examinations represent a challenge, similar to that posed by many other tasks in human life. Every new job, every new assignment, every new patient in a psychologist's office, every new trial for a lawyer, represents a challenge.

Children need guidance that enables them to respond to challenges in a rational manner so they neither overestimate nor overconfidently underestimate the potential dangers and attempt the task unprepared. Underestimation of dangers may be more harmful than overestimation; it is better to be overprepared than underprepared for a test in school or any other task.

Rational fear is based on a correct evaluation of potential dangers and one's own resources. If the dangers are indeed overwhelming, there is no point in entering the contest. If they are considerable but can be mastered with proper self-discipline and mobilization of resources, they offer a challenge and children should be encouraged to pursue the chance for victorious effort. Still, they should not be pushed to attempt impossible tasks or attend classes that are far too advanced for them. They should be given adequate encouragement to try for the best possible results and taught to take all the necessary steps to assure success.

Should a child fail after honest effort, he must not be punished for failing. He or she should never be told, "I told you so" but praised for honest effort and advised in a rational and encouraging manner how to prevent future errors.

Some parents tend to compare their children to other children—usually unfavorably. "Look, Mary, at your cousin Lucy. She is two months younger than you, and she got As in all her subjects. Aren't you ashamed of yourself? Why can't you get the same marks as Lucy?"

This kind of cruel comparison turns the child's normal and rational fear of tests and exams into a self-destructive anxiety. Poor Mary knows very well that her cousin is more gifted and nothing can be done about it. Her parents' remarks sound like accusations, and she perceives them as such and may blame herself for not being as smart as her cousin Lucy. She may believe that it is her fault she was born an average girl who gets B's and C's in school and think she should study harder so as not to disappoint and embarrass her parents.

The more upset she becomes and the more she fears parental disapproval, the less efficient her study will be. She may feel discouraged from making any effort because she knows she cannot be at the top of her class. Severe anxiety so paralyzes her that when she is taking a test, her mind goes blank.

SECTION 46. *Fear of the Unfamiliar and Strange*

The fear of the strange and unfamiliar has obvious survival value. An innate reaction, common to all human beings and several animal species, this fear serves an adaptive function, for it helps one to mobilize one's resources in the face of an unpredictable and potentially dangerous situation.

Most people, children and adults alike, have an ambivalent attitude toward the unknown. They feel secure with the familiar, but the unfamiliar tempts and repels at the same time. It is tempting to try a new kind of food, to see an unknown show, to travel to an unknown country and meet new and interesting people. All this may be very enjoyable provided one's feelings of security is not threatened. The success of risk taking depends on a correct estimate of one's own power. Too many people *think* they would like to travel to a war-torn country, climb to the top of a volcano, meet celebrated gangsters, or subject themselves to the exotic customs of a strange land—only to find the experience itself overwhelmingly frightening. Young and inexperienced drivers sometimes take unwarranted risks because their estimate of their reflexes and driving skills is unrealistic. Good skiers, seasoned mountain climbers, and shrewd businessmen take calculated risks in the field of their competence.

A small child has little or no experience in coping with dangers; thus his fear of the unknown may be a justified and wise method of dealing with the hazards of living. It is wrong to force a child to venture into the world prematurely. Instead he should be gradually taught to cope with the unknown and the unfamiliar.

The best method of coping with fear of the strange and unfamiliar is to make it no longer strange and unfamiliar. For instance, if a child fears his mirror reflection, the parent should hold the child's hand and play with him in front of the mirror. Later on the child himself will make faces and pull his tongue in front of the mirror.

Little children need instant reassurance, and a frightened infant should be calmed by holding him, patting, rocking, and so on. Older children should be gradually and patiently helped to get acquainted with objects and situations they fear.

If a child fears vacuum cleaners, for instance, the patient parent may disconnect the vacuum cleaner, touch it, and show it to him. If elevators cause alarm, the parent should enter the elevator with the child and show him how to press the buttons. On a trip in the mountains the parent should hold the frightened child's hand and help him up the slopes. Similarly, the parent should lead the child by the hand into a dark room; or she should pet the new cat or dog in the child's presence and allow him to get acquainted with the pet gradually.

Fears can be allayed or aggravated by pleasant or unpleasant experiences. A friendly and cheerful parental attitude can make fears disappear. A child who fears heights may get to like hiking trips in the mountains when he feels

CHILDREN' FEARS

loved and protected, when his parents enjoy the trip and enjoy his company. Needless to say, a child must not be exposed to dangerous and painful experiences that will greatly aggravate his fear. A child bitten by a dog, stranded in the mountains, caught in an elevator, or hurt in a dark room needs more time and many more pleasant experiences in similar situations to overcome his fears. With older children verbal explanation combined with a corrective experience is advisable, but verbal explanation alone may not suffice.

Familiar objects tend to reduce fears. A one- or two-year-old may be less afraid of strangers if he is allowed to suck his very familiar own thumb in their presence. Children who fear to go to sleep get a great deal of reassurance if their favorite teddy bear or a familiar piece of wool (security blanket) goes to bed with them. Traveling with little children can be enjoyable if the parents bring to the new and unknown hotel environment some pieces of the old and familiar environment, such as the child's favorite toys.

SECTION 47. *Fear of Vacuum Cleaners*

Loud noises and rapid movements evoke fear in practically all children. This fear is innate and never completely disappears, though it gradually diminishes with age.

When a two-year-old girl who feared vacuum cleaners was taken by her parents to visit her grandmother, she asked about the grandmother's vacuum cleaner. The grandmother, who knew of the little girl's fears, answered with a cute smile, "My vacuum cleaner went to the closet. He is tired and taking a nap."

The grandmother was proud of her story, but the frightened child broke into tears. "Couldn't a sleepy vacuum cleaner get up and walk around? And then, what would happen? Would he start his mean tricks again?"

One should not fan a child's fantasy; television producers do enough psychological harm with their frightening programs (see Section 53). Children tend to ascribe human traits to engines and inanimate nature in general, and rational parents should gradually help the child to see the world as it really is (See Section 48 on imaginary fears).

SECTION 48. *Imaginary Fears*

Some imaginary fears stem from the child's inadequate cognitive abilities. Overheard parental conversations are often misinterpreted. For instance, parental talk about famine in Bangladesh, riots in Ireland, or kidnappings in Italy may make the child think there is an imminent threat to himself and his family. Sometimes parents say frightening things in the presence of a child as if he or she does not exist or is deaf.

Most children's imaginary fears, however, stem from their own mental development. Children are prone to ascribe human traits to animals and inanimate nature, and often create imaginary beings and forces, some of them well-wishing and benevolent, some of them hostile and malevolent.

Children should be allowed to be children, and must not be prematurely forced to think and act like adults. Insisting on mental precocity simply does not work; sometimes it even causes considerable harm to the child's mental health. Deliberately slowing down the process of growth and maturation does not do any good to the child's mental health either.

Children go through certain developmental phases, and wise parents and teachers can greatly contribute to a smooth transition to a wholesome adulthood. A child must not be prevented from playing with an imaginary playmate or building castles out of blocks or reading *The Wizard of Oz* or *Gulliver's Travels*. However, the parents themselves should always retain their objective and factual judgment. Whenever asked, they should make it clear that witches, bogeys, monsters, and so on do not exist in life but only in stories. Parents must not regress nor infantilize themselves in the mistaken belief that this helps their children; their main task is to help children to grow up, and a correct perception of the world is of the utmost importance of normal functioning.

Every intelligent parent knows that a realistic perception of oneself and the world is the most important factor in mental health. People who distort reality, who underestimate or overestimate themselves or others, who exaggerate or misconstrue facts, who don't see things as they are, are not well adjusted. Mentally disturbed people experience extreme distortions of reality, and the most seriously disturbed suffer delusions and hallucinations.

Under no circumstances should parents encourage excessive fantasy in children. They should never threaten the child with bogeymen, ghosts, monsters, or any other supernatural creatures, nor ascribe human traits to inanimate objects such as vacuum cleaners or dishwashers. Such parental utterances give credence to the child's figments of imagination and perpetuate morbid fears.

Neither should children be ridiculed for having childish fears and fantasies. Making firm distinctions between imaginary and real things will help the child to get rid of his fears of nonexisting threats.

SECTION 49. *Lack of Fear*

Some parents overprotect their children. Motivated by their own anxiety and feelings of inadequacy, they take excessive care of their child. Even in adolescence they dress and undress their "baby"; they don't allow him to work in the summer; they will not send him away "alone" to camp; they encourage him to cling to them as if he were an infant.

An overprotected child gets the feeling that he will always be taken care of, and all his wishes and whims will be met forever. In such an atmosphere he develops a false feeling of security. Normally the two main factors of security are one's own power and self-confidence, and the presence of trustworthy and loyal allies (parents and later peers). Overprotection deprives the child of the opportunity to develop faith in his own powers. He relies on parental assurances that he'll always be well taken care of and develops an infantile-parasitic attitude.

I have treated several people of this kind in psychoanalytic psychotherapy. One of them did brazen things as a child and adolescent, sure that his good parents would always bail him out. He grew up sadly unprepared to cope with adult life and often behaved like a spoiled, selfish, inconsiderate, and thoughtless child.

Quite often adolescents simulate lack of fear and disdain for danger. Usually this bravado is fostered by group spirit and peer culture. The "old generation" is judged to be cowardly and conservative, while "youth" is believed to have great ideas and earth-shaking innovations.

Adolescent lack of fear is often a cover-up for feelings of inadequacy (see Section 38 on fear of sex). Adolescents are no longer children but they are not yet adults. They resent being treated as children, and often believe that pretending to have more power than they actually have will convince their parents and teachers—and, above all, their peers—that they are fearless individuals.

Tactful parents do not dampen adolescent enthusiasm or provoke unnecessary conflicts. They relate to their adolescent sons and daughters in a friendly, unpatronizing manner. They keep a tab on reality and, whenever necessary, point out to the adolescent existing dangers. They do not preach but are ready to give sober and encouraging advice.

SECTION 50. *Nightmares or Night Terrors*

Most dreams represent the fulfillment of forbidden, repressed, or rejected wishes, and some of them reflect vehement inner conflicts. Nightmares convey the frightening thought that a horrifying wish may come true.

Severe punishment is the most frequent theme of nightmares. The punishment is usually related to the child's sexual and/or aggressive impulses. Many children harbor in their unconscious death wishes toward competing siblings, frustrating parents, punitive teachers, or anyone who might hurt them. Children are afraid to admit to themselves their hostile wishes, but the wishes cannot be denied altogether and so they disrupt sleep.

Most children masturbate and have incestuous sexual fantasies. The best way of handling this is not to handle it at all. Certainly there is no reason for recrimination or punishment for having normal sexual cravings (see Sections 12 and 38).

A child punished for masturbation or threatened with punishment may control himself and refrain from masturbation during waking hours. But as soon as he falls asleep the unconscious wishes may come up and the child may dream about playing with his or her genitalia. This may arouse severe anxiety and a gorilla, monster, or Nazi henchman may threaten in the dream to cut off his penis or hurt him or her in some other way.

Even more frightening are nightmares related to aggressive impulses. In many cases sleep disturbances, nightmares, and night terrors call for professional help. Should the child volunteer to communicate the content of his nightmares, parents should not play psychoanalyst and try to interpret his unconscious. Simple reassurance often allays fears temporarily but may not suffice to prevent the recurrence of frightening dreams.

When a child wakes up in terror from a nightmare a sympathetic mother may pick him up and put him in her bed. Obviously this is most comforting, but in the long run it is a reward that *encourages* nightmares. From then on the nightmares will serve a dual purpose: bring punishment for forbidden wishes (the dream itself) and secure gratification of a hidden wish (sleeping with mother). Thus the kind and loving mother nicely contributes to the child's confusion by infantilizing him and facilitating his regression to a lower developmental level. No child should be allowed to sleep with his mother.

A frightened child needs loving reassurance that will help him to outgrow his fears. It is counterproductive to force him to overcome his fears by prodding, threatening, or punishing.

SECTION 51. *Phobias*

Sometimes a child unconsciously substitutes one fear for another, especially when the initial fear creates inner conflict and guilt. For instance, a ten-year-old girl who feared and hated her irritable and explosive mother developed a fear of cats. Her mother's name was Catherine and her husband called her Kitty. The little girl's fear of cats was less severe than her fear that she might hurt her mother.

Another child who felt like stealing, and who had already stolen some money from her mother's purse, developed an excessive fear of burglars. This substitute fear was socially acceptable and created no inner conflict, while the original fear of her own dishonest impulses produced profound anxiety combined with the fear of severe punishment.

While the child fears to disclose his real fear, he unconsciously wishes to get rid of the burdensome conflict. He may be perplexed by nightmares in which he is subjected to severe punishment. He may wish to share his discomforting feelings with someone he trusts, and patiently listening and understanding parents might be his first choice. Understanding parents may alleviate the child's fear and enable him to confess and confide, and resolve the conflict that underlies his fears and possibly overcome the fear itself. (See Chapter I.)

SECTION 52. School Phobia

Children may refuse to go to school for a variety of reasons. In many cases the avoidance of school is caused by harsh and unfair teachers, the fear of being hurt and/or ridiculed by schoolmates, or the fear of scholastic failure and resulting parental punishment.

A truant is a child who habitually avoids school; he runs away from school. Some children do not run *away* from school but run *toward* something that alleviates their anxiety.

Phobic children "run home" to mother. They are afraid to be away from home because they worry that something may happen when they are gone. They may develop headaches, bellyaches, nausea, dizziness, and other psychosomatic symptoms to justify their insistence on staying home with mother. Phobic children are not malingerers or liars—their headaches are real and they actually do throw up. Their symptoms develop unconsciously, and they cannot be blamed for feelings and symptoms that are beyond their control.

It is worth stressing that the majority of children with school phobia do well in school. Apparently they do not fear scholastic failure but *separation* and *abandonment*. Some children who recently witnessed a death in the family are prone to school phobia. They feel their presence at home can prevent bad things (death) from happening. A death in the family or illness rarely causes school phobia in a child who is otherwise well adjusted. Such traumatic events precipitate the phobia in children who are susceptible.

School phobia has a variety of causes. Sometimes it grows slowly and gradually develops as a by-product of the child's deep-rooted anxiety that makes him cling to the protective home environment. Sometimes it is produced by a faulty parent-child relationship.

Some anxious mothers fear being home alone. As the husband must leave the house to go to work, the wife resorts to her child for company. She may not admit this to herself—as a rule, she is not fully aware of her wish—but she never misses the opportunity to "allow" her child to skip school on rainy days or when he or she sneezes or scratches a finger. In many instances the child empathizes (senses) the mother's wish and makes his own excuses for not going to school.

Just as frequent, and psychologically more serious, is the school phobia caused by the child's worry that something horrible may happen to mother and/or father in his absence. Normally parents are perceived by their children as being strong and friendly and dependable (see Chapter VIII). But when one or both of the parents display true or imaginary illnesses, confide in and complain to the child—in short, present themselves as weak and despondent creatures—in a reversal of roles the child may worry about his parents instead of them worrying about him. In extreme cases this kind of relationship can play havoc with the child's mental health.

Inconsistent and insecure parents may give the child the impression that *they* fear separation, that *they* need the child's presence. Their unconscious clinging to the child discourages his or her independence and self-assertiveness. Many overdependent and overprotected children develop school phobia, as if they sense the need behind their mother's solicitude for them. Of course, consciously every mother wishes her child to go to school and be independent and outgoing, but unconscious anxieties may make her act in an inconsistent manner that, in turn, fans the child's anxiety and overdependence.

Some parents unwittingly and unwillingly reinforce their child's school phobia by paying too much attention to the child's complaints of headaches, nausea, or bellyaches, many of which may be psychosomatic. Certainly any pain, true or imaginary, requires parental attention, and the complaints warrant medical examination. The suffering child should be taken to a doctor, but *before or after school hours*. Taking the child to a doctor during school hours encourages his staying home from school.

It is advisable to pay as little attention as possible to a phobic child's physical complaints. An extra dose of sympathy by an anxious mother will only aggravate the symptoms. A friendly, firm, encouraging, but not permissive and certainly not pitying attitude can help the child. A frank conversation may be necessary, and in some cases the child should be referred for brief psychotherapy to a competent child clinical psychologist, psychiatrist, or psychoanalyst.

Section 53. *Television-induced Fears*

Many childhood fears are caused by watching terror scenes on TV. Children take television seriously and be-

161

CHILDREN'S FEARS IN ALPHABETICAL ORDER

lieve that the actors who perform violent scenes are not acting and that the screen represents real happenings. Every so often children develop serious states of anxiety fanned, and often caused by what they saw on TV. Scientific research has found that children who watch TV a great deal are more anxious and suffer from more and more severe fears than children who spend little time in front of the television with its crime and horror stories.

After watching violent scenes on TV many a child is afraid to go to sleep. If all this is true, as the child believes, how can he be sure that the violence he has seen will not be directed against him and his family?

Scientific studies show that many TV programs educate preadolescents and adolescents in violent behavior. Even greater harm is caused to younger children, who take the TV shows literally and watch violent programs with crippling horror.

There is no doubt that violence on television not only increases fears but also reduces inhibitions against aggressive behavior. Several articles on aggression in the *International Encyclopedia of Psychiatry, Psychology, Psychoanalysis, & Neurology* present objective and conclusive evidence that younger children become frightened and develop sleep disturbances and nightmares, while older children and adolescents become uninhibited in their antisocial behavior. Lack of fear (see Section 49) is no less abnormal than excessive fear; both lead to abnormal behavior.

Some juvenile delinquents who commit crimes of violence have been "brainwashed" by frequent and prolonged viewing of TV violence. Many spend several hours everyday watching crime programs, such as "Kojak," "Baretta," and "Starsky and Hutch."

Violence on television teaches children that one can get away with murder. To some of them, pulling a trigger becomes as common as killing a fly. By the age of eighteen

CHILDREN'S FEARS

American youngsters have spent eleven thousand hours in schools, but they have watched eighteen thousand TV murders!

The vast majority of children, who do not feel compelled to attack innocent people after watching TV, instead begin to believe that they themselves are an easy target for kidnappers, gangsters, and murderers. After all, on television criminals are everywhere and attack with impunity. Small wonder that many children feel insecure even in their own home and develop severe anxiety.

Bibliography

Abraham, K., *Selected Papers,* New York, Basic Books, 1954.

Bowlby, J., *Attachment and Loss,* New York, Basic Books, 1973.

Freud, S., *Standard Edition of the Complete Psychological Works,* London, The Hogarth Pres Ltd., 1963, Vol. 16.

Jersild, A. T., *Child Psychology,* New York, Prentice Hall, 1974.

Murphy, L. B., *The Widening World of Childhood,* New York, Basic Books, 1962.

Sullivan, H. S., *Conceptions of Modern Psychiatry,* Washington, D.C., White Foundation, 1947.

Index

INDEX

INDEX

INDEX